# MICROENCAPSULATION

*Processes and Applications*

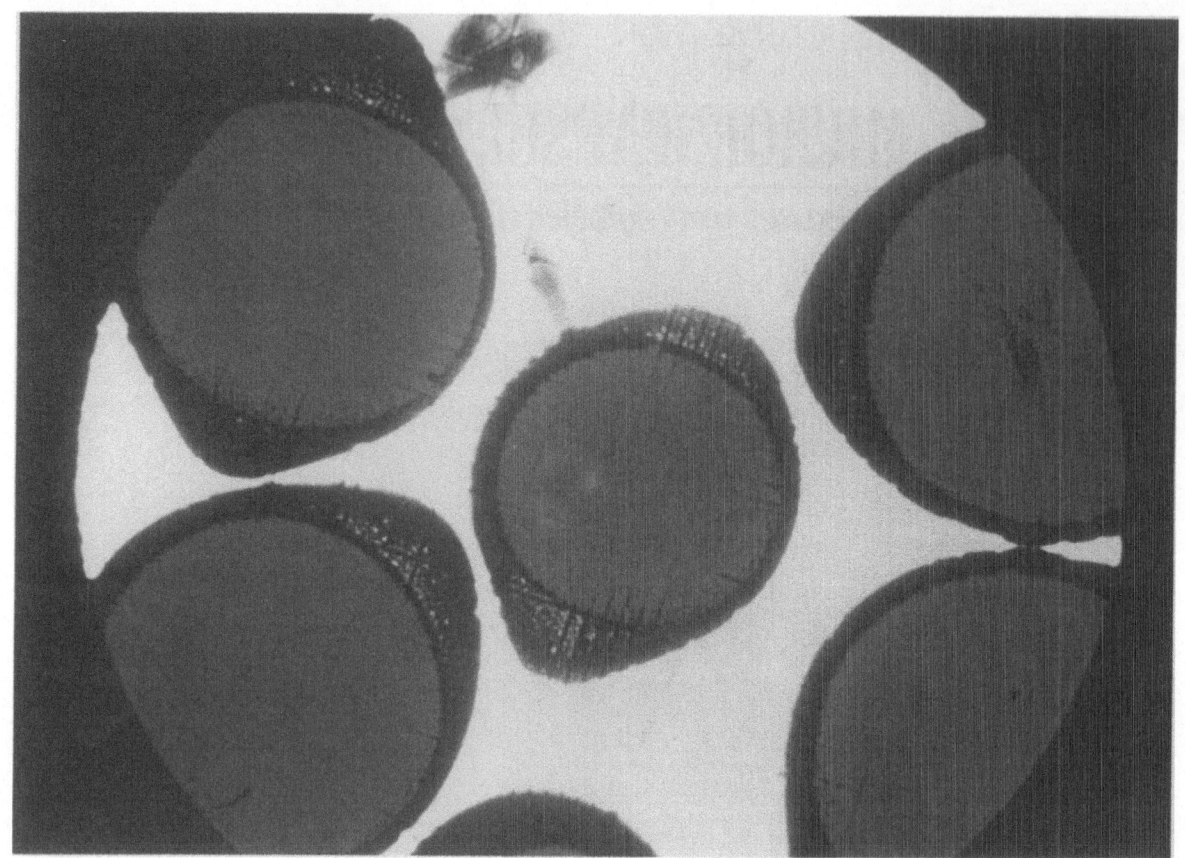

Gelatin microcapsule containing oil core

# MICROENCAPSULATION

## Processes and Applications

Edited by
## Jan E. Vandegaer

PLENUM PRESS • NEW YORK AND LONDON

Library of Congress Cataloging in Publication Data

American Chemical Society Symposium on Microencapsulation: Processes
  and Applications, Chicago, 1973.
  Microencapsulation: processes and applications.

  Includes bibliographical references.
  1. Microencapsulation—Congresses. I. Vandegaer, Jan E., 1927-      ed.
II. American Chemical Society. III. Title.
TS198.C33A43      1973                    660.2'842                    74-6125

ISBN-13: 978-1-4684-0741-9      e-ISBN-13: 978-1-4684-0739-6
DOI: 10.1007/978-1-4684-0739-6

Proceedings of the American Chemical Society Symposium on
Microencapsulation: Processes and Applications
held in Chicago, August 28, 1973

# INTRODUCTION

Jan E. Vandegaer*

My co-chairmen, Mr. Herman Nack and Dr. Wade Van Valkenburg, and I believe that the present symposium volume, despite its brevity, ranges across the entire spectrum of microencapsulation research and achieves a fair balance between the different techniques of microencapsulation and the many applications to which these techniques are aimed. According to my classification, one can distinguish here between physical processes, chemical processes, and mechanical processes.

Among the physical processes I consider the coacervation technique first developed by the researchers of the National Cash Register Company. Here the polymer simply undergoes a physical change by precipitation on a droplet interface and is later chemically hardened. This process is represented by several papers in this symposium. For instance, professor S. Kubo speaks on the liquid crystal containing light sensitive microcapsules made by coacervation. Encapsulated vegetable fats in cattle feeds is the subject of Dr. J. Bitman and his coworkers of the U. S. Department of Agriculture. Dr. Thies and his coworkers formerly from the National Cash Register Company speak on the liquid extractions carried out with microcapsule packed columns. Here also the capsules were prepared with a variation of the coacervation technique. Dr. Luzzi and his coworkers of the University of Georgia speak on the encapsulation of spherical particles as a characteristic of gelatin fractions.

Among the predominantly chemical microencapsulation processes where the capsule wall is formed in situ by a chemical polymerization reaction we have the interfacial condensation polymerization method represented by a contribution from Professor T.M.S. Chang

*Address correspondence c/o Plenum Publishing Corporation, 227 W. 17th St., New York, N. Y. 10011.

of McGill University of Montreal, Canada, who talks about artificial cells prepared from semipermeable microcapsules. Also illustrative of this method is a contribution on microencapsulated pesticides by C. B. Desavigny and E. E. Ivy of Pennwalt Corporation. Another method of polymerization in situ is microencapsulation by vapor deposition, the subject of W. M. Jayne of Union Carbide Corporation.

The more mechanical methods of microencapsulation are represented by two techniques, one involving a fluidized bed the other involving mainly a centrifugal method. The fluidized bed method is covered in a paper by H. Hall and T. M. Hinkes of the Wisconsin Alumini Research Foundation. The centrifugal and other related methods are treated by Mr. J. E. Goodwin and Mr. Sommerville of the Southwest Research Institute of San Antonio, Texas.

Dr. G. Baxter of Moore Business Forms, studied capsules made by mechanical methods as well as by chemical methods. Mr. Russell G. Arnold of the Bureau of Veteranary Medicine of the Food and Drug Administration draws our attention to the procedures to be used for securing approval of a new animal drug application for the marketing of microencapsulated products. And last but not least, we have a contribution by Mr. G. O. Fanger on "Microencapsulation a Brief History and Introduction, whose title speaks for itself.

The above papers were all presented at the symposium of the Division of Organic Coatings and Plastics Chemistry of the American Chemical Society at the 166th meeting of the ACS in Chicago held from August 26 to 31 in 1973. At the request of the publisher I have taken the liberty of adding another chapter to this book describing in somewhat fundamental detail the principles behind the encapsulation by coacervation.

Our Symposium covers a wide range of applications. One contribution from the Wisconsin Alumni Research Foundation deals primarily with pharmaceutical applications while two other ones deal with applications in the graphic arts field. Agricultural applications involve microencapsulated pesticides and encapsulated vegetable fats in cattle feeds. Catalyst activity control is one application of microencapsulation by vapor deposition. Separation techniques are covered by three papers; one of them describes a separation of amines carried out on microcapsule-packed columns. Another one describes use of activated charcoal as the scavenging agent inside the microcapsules. This paper and a third one by Professor Chang deal with biochemical applications of these microcapsules as used in separation techniques. As one can readily see this short symposium covers a variety of applications in different fields.

And this brings us really to the crux of the problem of dealing with microencapsulation in any systematic way.  Such a large variety of techniques and scientific disciplines come into play in the manufacture of microcapsules.  Furthermore the fields of applications are as wide as the human imagination.  In almost any place where microreservoirs are needed or can be visualized these techniques-or at least one of them- may suggest themselves. The proposed need for the microreservoirs may be protection during incorporation for safety or other reasons; it may be for release triggered later or sustained over a longer period as desired with certain pesticides.  The reason may be controlled activity of certain chemical agents such as catalysts.  Or it may be the extremely large surface to volume ratio which is desirable in highly efficient and fast chemical exchanges.  In yet other applications the need for microencapsulation exists because one wants to protect ingredients during certain processes.  An example is presented here in this symposium where encapsulated vegetable fats are microencapsulated in cattle feed for reason of protection in the cow's rumen where they would normally be hydrogenated by microorganisms.

Since microencapsulation covers such a great variety of engineering techniques and scientific disciplines in the manufacture of the capsules and such a wide variety of potential fields of application, it makes it extremely difficult to present a systematic view of the total effort being dispensed in this field. It also makes it very difficult for anybody new to the art who has a potential application in mind to make a meaningful start in this complex field.  One could point here to many false starts undertaken in this field ending in frustrating results.  All too often it happened in the past that a potential user of microencapsulation technology started out by not thoroughly thinking through the potential problems of the final application.  He also quite often approached a processor who with his specific process could not possibly make the capsules which would most efficiently perform in the intended application.  Therefore let me use the space in this introduction to counsel new users of microencapsulation technology when first contemplating a microencapsulation application they should attempt to become thoroughly acquainted not only with the potential but also the pitfalls and limitations of each chemical, physical, and mechanical method in order to better choose which one among these is best suited for the intended application.

We hope that this volume may assist potential users to choose the proper microencapsulation techniques for their intended use.

The editor wishes to express his thanks to all the authors and their respective organizations who contributed to the symposium and to this volume.  He wishes especially to express his

gratitude to his co-chairmen Dr. J. Wade Van Valkenburg and
especially Mr. Herman Mack who made most of the initial contacts
with the authors of this volume.  Finally he wishes to express
appreciation of the assistance of Drs. P. Readio and R. Kent who
were most helpful in the editing of this volume and whose layman's
view of the new field of encapsulation was most appreciated.

# CONTENTS

MICROENCAPSULATION

A BRIEF HISTORY AND INTRODUCTION

Gene O. Fanger

Ball Corporation/Technical Division

Muncie, Indiana  47302

## Introduction

A number of excellent reviews have been published on microencapsulation (I-XI).  It is not the purpose of this paper to give
a comprehensive review of the field, but rather to acquaint the
listener with the historical background and give him a general
appreciation of the capabilities and limitation of the technology.

Microencapsulation began with the creation of a living cell.
Most one-celled plants or animals are living examples of the
wonders of microencapsulation.  These natural capsular membranes
are remarkably successful in fulfilling specific functions.  Among
the most important functions are protection of the interior
material (core) and control of the flow of materials (permeation)
across the cell membrane.  Because of their outer protection,
plant seeds and bacteria spores have remained viable for periods
of over 100 years (1).  Black pigmentation within the walls protect fungii spores in hostile environments by screening out
sunlight (2).  Charged lipid bilayers often act as permeability
valves.  Permeability of water through cytoplasmic membranes may
be $10^{10}$ times larger than the permeability of ions (3).  Even a
chicken egg has been engineered with a protective wall, thick
enough to provide maximum protection during incubation, and still
thin enough to allow breakage at the moment of hatching.

## Historical

One man's attempt at copying nature began in a Dayton, Ohio
laboratory.  In the late 30's, Barrett Green, a young chemist
just out of school, was intrigued by the dearth of information in

1

the colloid field on liquids dispersed in solids.  He had earlier
recognized the usefulness of such disperse systems in photographic
applications.  When his company needed a product that would give
multiple paper copies without carbon paper, Barrett Green turned
to his new ideas on dispersions.  By 1940 the first working no-
carbon-required paper had been prepared, but that was only the
beginning.  His breakthrough came in 1942 while he was investigating Bungenberg de Jong's coacervation studies (4,5).

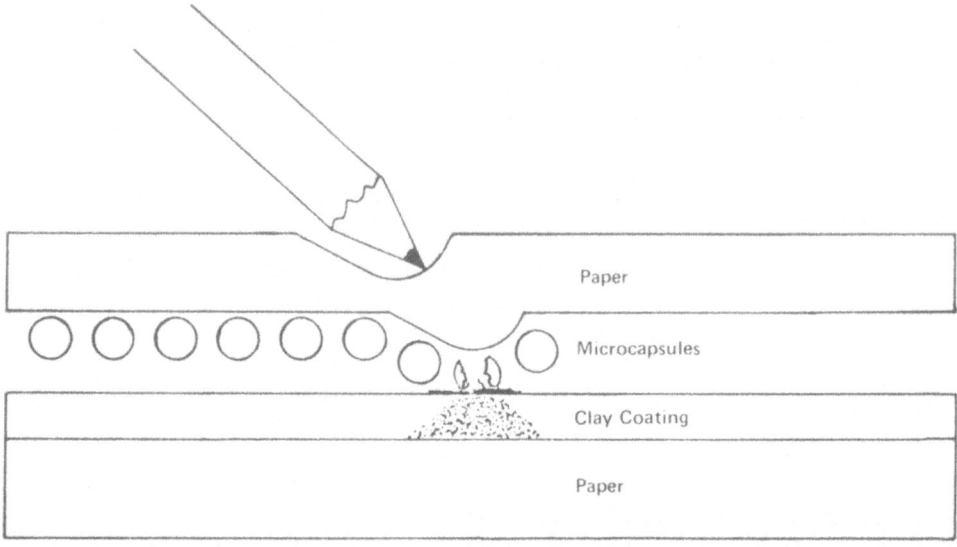

Figure 1.  *Pressure-activated release of encapsulated dye-precursor to give a color reaction on paper coated with acidic clay.*

One paper mentioned the preparation of solid gelatin spheres,
while another dealt with the inclusion of an oil phase within a
gelatin coacervate.  Mr. Green used both concepts and prepared
the first gelatin microcapsules.  From this crude beginning it
was nine long years to the development of a marketable product.
The new printing system was triggered by including a colorless
dye-base in the oil droplets and coating a second sheet of paper
with acidic clay (Figure 1).

Coacervation

Coacervates may be divided into two types: 1) simple and 2)
complex.  (See also chapter by J. Vandegaer)  The major difference

is the presence of a second (or even third) colloid in complex coacervation systems.

Coacervation can occur in solutions of colloids through the addition of inorganic salts, dilution, or temperature changes in the case of simple coacervation, and dilution, temperature, or pH changes in the case of complex coacervation.

Mr. Green used complex coacervation to prepare a colloid rich gelatin-gum arabic coacervate phase into which he dispersed droplets of a second oil phase (6,7,8). The chemistry of the wetting is such that the coacervate film wets and coats the oil droplets, and can then be hardened in place using crosslinking agents such as formaldehyde or gluteraldehyde (Figure 2).

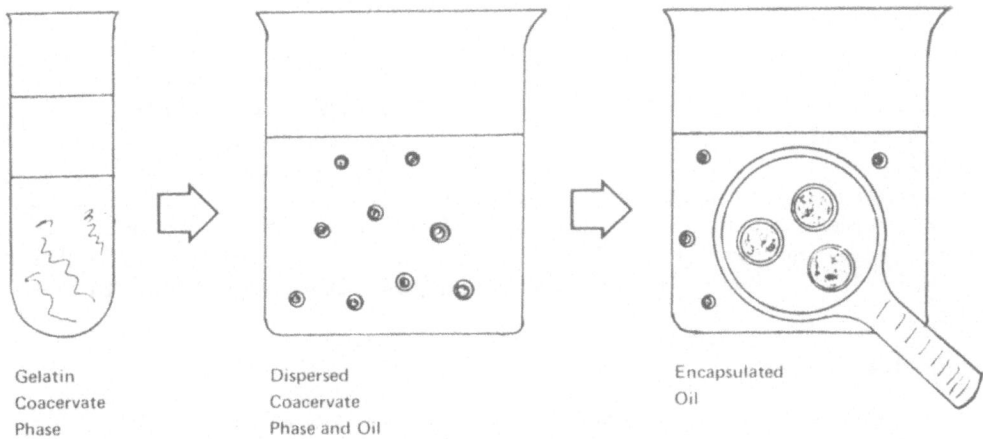

Gelatin
Coacervate
Phase

Dispersed
Coacervate
Phase and Oil

Encapsulated
Oil

*Figure 2.    Representation of encapsulation of oil droplet by gelatin coacervation.*

Later, improvements in encapsulation efficiency were achieved by including a third colloid capable of carrying greater surface charges(9-13).

Careful control of the drying process produced low-permeability capsules in which low-boiling oils could be held for extended periods of time. Since it was not possible to encapsulate polar liquids in a gelatin colloid wall directly, an alternative procedure was perfected whereby the interior oil core was exchanged with a polar liquid after the capsule shell had been prepared (14). A special post-treatment was often required to seal in the new polar core liquid (15).

As these processes were perfected, other uses were envisioned for the capsules. Products such as gasoline bricks, dry martini capsules, fragrance-releasing stationery, and water-cooled cigarettes found their way into the news.

Phase Separation

Once it was shown that aqueous solutions of gelatin could be utilized to contain organic solutions, someone asked, "Why not encapsulate aqueous solutions in organic materials?" In 1959, another laboratory in Dayton was set up to do just that. As a member of this group, I had a part in perfecting a new encapsulating technique using "phase separation" (16).

(Now polar liquids could be encapsulated directly inside of polymeric materials.) In this process a liquid "separated phase" was produced which could be made to wet and wrap polar substrates. This mobile coating was then hardened into a capsule using chemical or physical methods (17).

Together with some newer innovations in coacervation, the combined technology was focused on commercialization (18-22). Such products as pharmaceutical timed-release encapsulated analgesics (23), encapsulated liquid crystals (24), and adhesive capsules used in space exploration resulted (25). Scientists at other companies were also making major contributions to our knowledge and extending the utilization of this science (26-29). Commercial products based on microencapsulation are shown in Figure 3.

Dehydration

At about the same time the NCR group was studying coacervation, a group of scientists led by Dr. Marco Cannalonga at Hoffman La Roche were investigating various ways of protecting vitamins from premature decomposition. Using Taylor's earlier work as a starting point (30), they found that by emulsifying an oil phase containing vitamins in an aqueous coating solution and atomizing it into fine droplets, new dehydration techniques could be utilized to produce solid powders containing active vitamins with increased long-term stability (31).

Another dehydration technique utilized a hydroscopic liquid polymer or solvent to remove water from the coating and achieve a solid dry capsule film (32,33). Various other dehydration techniques have also been used to form capsules (34,35).

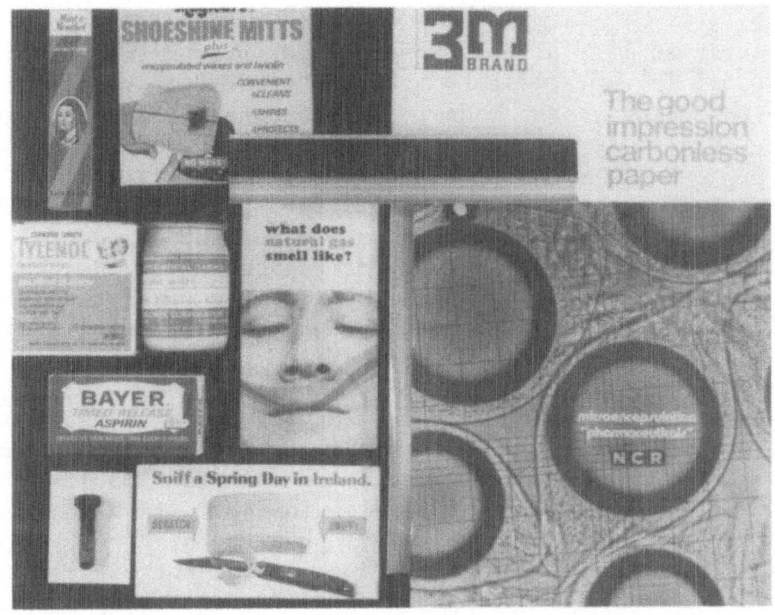

Figure 3. Commercial products using microencapsulation.

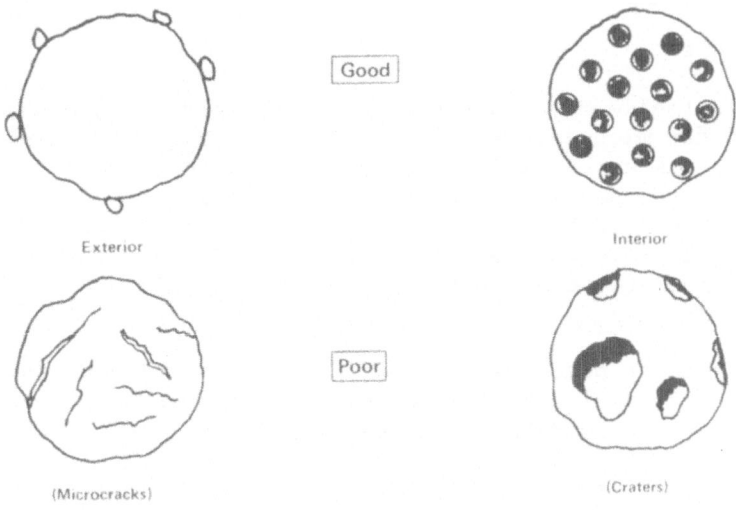

Figure 4. Representation of spray-dried microcapsules.

Spray Drying

As early as 1927 A. Bolk Roberts had spray dried emulsions
of flavor oil in gum acadia to prepare "Drydex" capsules (X).
Over the following years, modest improvements were made in gum
acacia-spray dried encapsulation (36).

Then, in the early 50's technological advances led to the
commercial drying of milk, coffee, and other food products.  These
advances, along with the discovery of a process for the preparation of water-soluble dextrin (37), opened the way for spray
drying flavor or fragrance oil microcapsules of greater stability
and containing higher oil levels (38-42).

Considering the fact that spray drying requires heat to
remove large volumes of water from the coating solution, amazing
achievements have been made in capturing volatile liquids within
a solid matrix and stabilizing them against oxidative and thermal
degradation.  In contrast to capsules prepared by coacervation
and phase separation, spray dried capsules are not single droplet
capsules, but instead are composed of hundreds of tiny dispersed
oil droplets in a water-soluble polymer matrix.  A representation
is shown in Figure 4.

Out of this humble beginning has emerged a multimillion
dollar business in spray dried microcapsules, particularly useful
to the food and cosmetic industries (43).

Fluidized Bed

At Battelle Memorial Institute fluidized bed technology was
tailored for microencapsulation.  Either a liquid coating solution
or molten wax could be sprayed onto fluidized solid core particles
to form microcapsules.  Alternatively, liquids could be included
in the process if they were first frozen to a solid form.  In
addition, a fluidized bed of meltable coating material could be
used to instantly coat molten core droplets falling into it
(44,45).  Figure 5.

Because of problems in particle agglomeration during coating,
and difficulties in fluidizing powders composed of very small
particles, the fluid bed technique was limited to capsules of 200

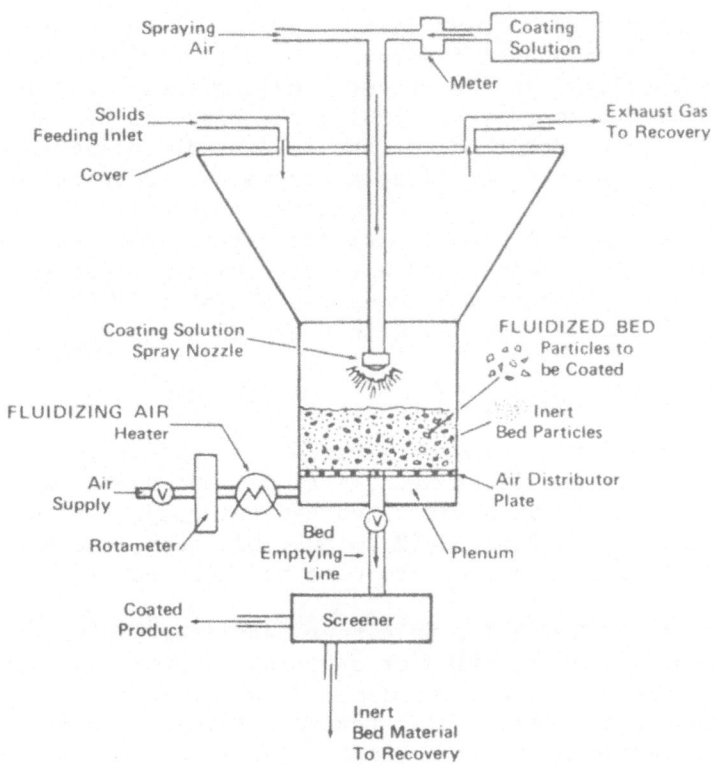

*Figure 5.    Fluidized bed coating.  Nack, H., U.S. Patent 3,382,093 (May 1968).*

microns and larger. However, by incorporating a deagglomeration
jet, designed specifically for coating particles in the 5 to 200
micron size range, smaller capsules have been prepared and used in
pharmaceutical products (46).

## Chemical Vapor Deposition

Though as yet not commercialized, C.V.D. techniques applied
to the coating of high-melting metallic particles have produced
interesting results. In one process nuclear fuel particles have
been coated with carbon by condensing the products of the thermal
decomposition of hydrocarbons on the suspended, moving core
particles (47). Another utilizes a plasma jet to vaporize the
reactants for the coating and a fluidized bed to provide means for
condensing the reactant vapors onto the particle surface (48).
Vacuum metallization techniques have also been applied to microencapsulation (49). Again, a lower capsule size limit in the order
of 200 microns can be expected with these techniques.

## Mechanical Methods

Microencapsulation drew on a variety of disciplines as it
developed. One of the first mechanical methods was that of
D. E. Wurster, who applied fluidized bed technology to the mechanical formation of capsules (50-52). Multiple seed coatings for
delayed germination have been produced by this technique (53).

Scientists at S.W.R.I., by either centrifugally forcing core
material through coating films or shooting it from gun-like tubes,
prepared a variety of new and unusual capsular products (54).
Even a technique harnessing electrostatic forces to coat aerosol
droplets was developed at IIT Research Institute (55-57). Develop-
ments at Western Reserve Laboratories led to an extrusion
technique currently used commercially in the preparation of flavor
oil capsules (58).

Dr. N. F. Cardarelli at the University of Akron incorporated
special organic materials into rubber pellets to produce "time-
release" capsules. Products based on this technique have been
useful in boicidal and environmental application (59-60).

Pan coating is a commonly used mechanical process for preparing macro-capsules (pills) in the pharmaceutical industry. It has
been adopted to the production of slow-releasing fertilizer by
scientists working at the T.V.A. labs(61). A number of other
mechanical methods of preparing capsules have been mentioned in
the literature (62-65).

In-Situ Polymerization

In-situ polymerization is a variation of chemical vapor deposition, in which the core particle can be either solid or
liquid and in which lower temperatures are generally employed.
In a National Lead Co. process, core particles are suspended in
toluene containing a Ziegler type catalyst, and ethylene gas is
then bubbled through the mixture. As the ethylene polymerizes on
the core particle, surface microcapsules are formed (66-67).

Dr. William Gorham and others at UCC developed another
process in which a cyclic di-p-xylylene is pyrolyzed to form
reactive diradicals which can be made .to polymerize on the surface
of moving core particles (68-70).

Both of the above processes have led to commercial products.
On the other hand a technique developed at Stanford Research
Institute for encapsulating aerosol particles by in-situ polymerization (71) and a glow discharge technique to generate ionized
organic monomer species developed by Radiation Research (72) are,
as yet, non-commercial.

Interfacial Polymerization and Membrane Properties

In 1959 DuPont researchers conducted a dramatic demonstra-
tion, at a national ACS meeting, in which nylon film was prepared
by interfacial polymerization (75). Following that meeting,
almost everyone in our field became interested in applying interfacial polymerization to microencapsulation.

The basic chemistry involved contacting an organic solution
of acid chloride with an aqueous solution of a diamine to produce
a film at the interface of the two liquids. If droplets of one
solution are added to the other or produced by stirring one solution into the other, microcapsules can be obtained. However, the
resulting capsules were more permeable than was desirable for
containment applications. Dr. Vandegaer got around this by including other crosslinking components in one of the reactive
solutions (77-80). Others decided to utilize the natural permeability of such capsules as useful capsular membranes. To
illustrate this potential, the permeability of nylon microcapsules
to a variety of organic molecules is shown in Figure 9. Some
groups became involved with investigating microcapsular membranes
as components of artificial organs (81-84). Others worked on
perfecting capsular systems tailored to counter specific metabolic
or biological deficiencies, such as hereditary enzyme defects
(86-87).

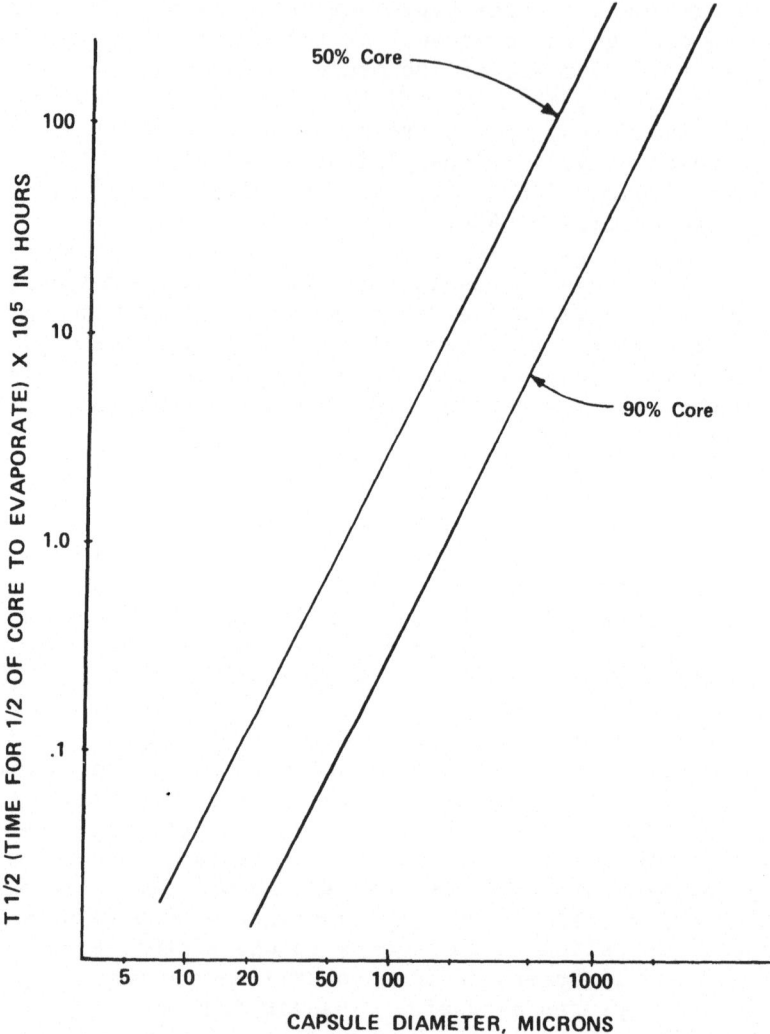

*Figure 6.*    *The effect of capsule size on evaporative core loss (encapsulated water in nitrocellulose).*

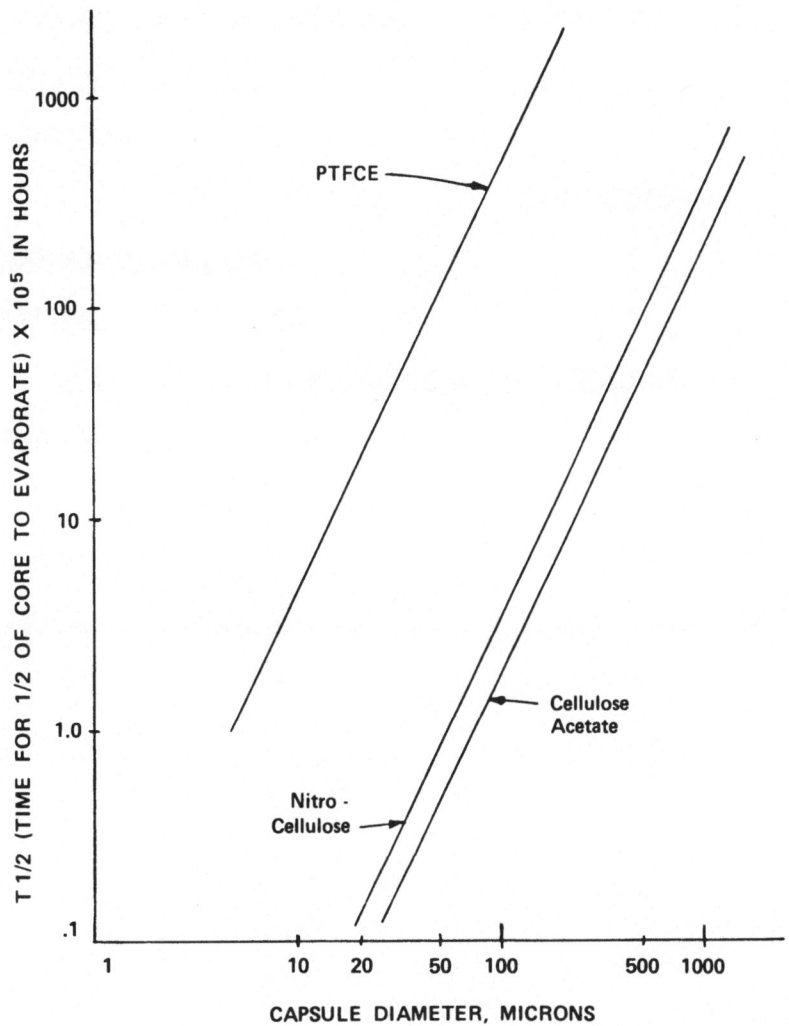

*Figure 7.    The influence of polymeric structure on evaporative core loss (50% core / 50% wall).*

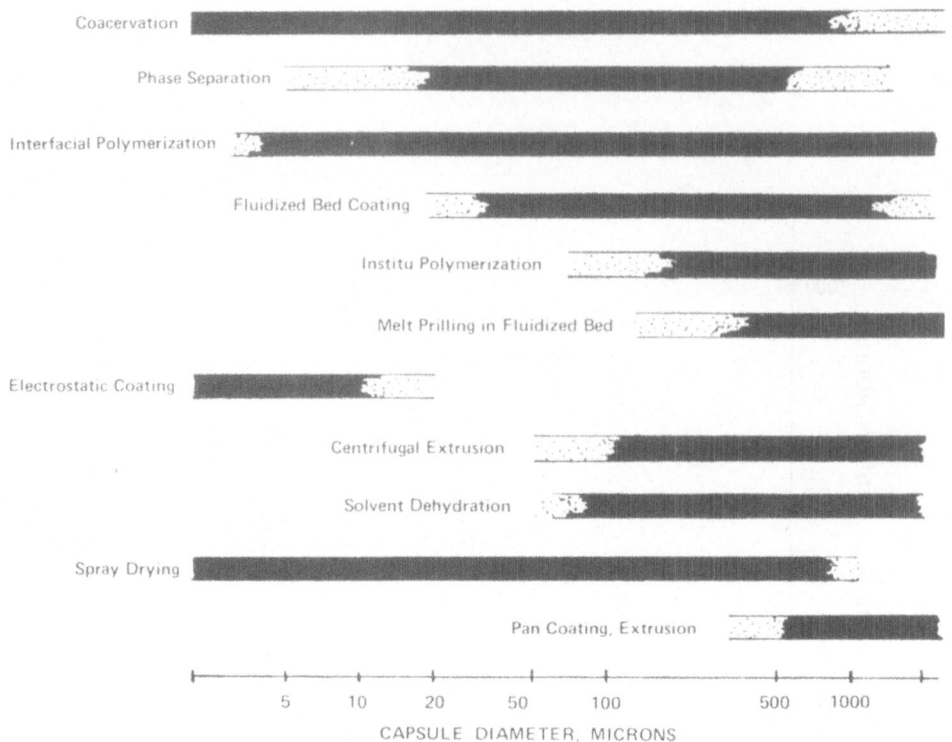

Figure 8.    *The range of capsule size produced in a variety of encapsulation processes.*

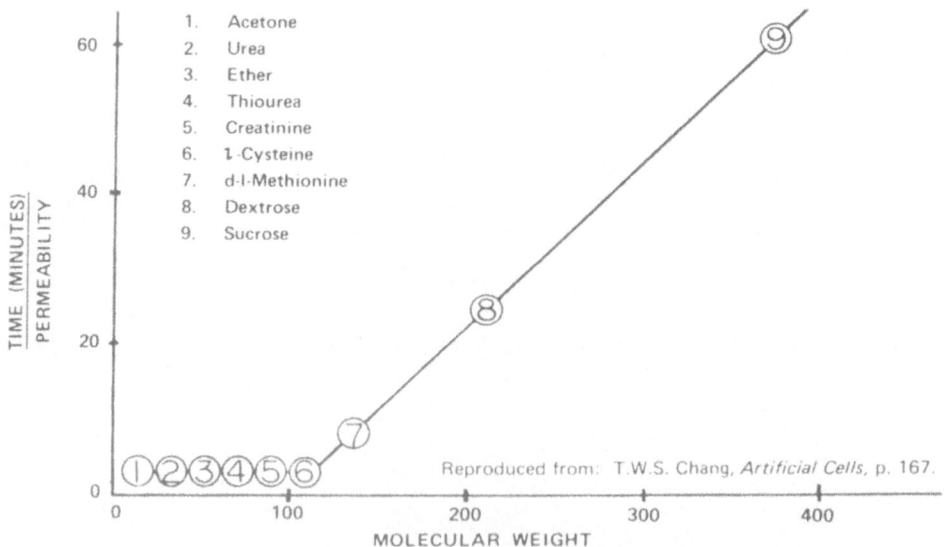

Figure 9.    *The permeability of nylon microcapsules.*

Table 1. *Choosing a Solvent Core Polymer Wall Capsular Combination Using Solubility Parameter Data (1, 2).*

| SOLVENT CORE | PARAMETER | CLASS | POLYMER WALL | PARAMETER | CLASS |
|---|---|---|---|---|---|
| A) Water | 23.4 | III | 1) Elvax 40 | 7.1-10.0 | II |
| B) Glycerol | 16.5 | III | 2) Gilsonite | 7.8- 8.5 | II |
| C) Ethanol | 12.7 | III | 3) Silicone DC-23 | 7.4- 7.8 | II |
| D) Butanol | 11.4 | III | 4) Hypalon 30 | 7.8- 8.5 | II |
| E) Ethylamine | 10.0 | III | 5) Rosin, WW | 7.4-10.8 | II |
| F) Acetaldehyde | 10.3 | II | 6) Geon 121 | 7.8- 9.9 | II |
| G) Methyl Ethyl Ketone | 9.3 | II | 7) Epon 864 | 8.5-14.7 | II |
| H) Ethyl Acrylate | 8.6 | II | 8) Piccoflex 120 | 9.3- 9.9 | II |
| I) Dioctyl Phthalate | 7.9 | II | 9) Polyester 49001 | 9.3- 9.9 | II |
| J) Diethyl Ether | 7.4 | II | 10) Ethyl Cellulose N-22 | 7.4-10.8 | II |
| K) Chloroform | 9.3 | I | 11) Bakelite BKL-2620 | 8.4-14.7 | II |
| L) Toluene | 8.9 | I | 12) Nitrocellulose RS | 7.8-14.7 | II |
| M) Turpentine | 8.1 | I | 13) Carbowax 4000 | 8.5-14.7 | II |
| N) Freon 22 | 7.6 | I | 14) Saran F-220 | 10.8-14.7 | II |
| O) n-Pentane | 7.0 | I | 15) Versalon 1112 | 9.5-11.4 | III |
| | | | 16) Nylon, Type 8 | 11.9-14.5 | III |

(1)     A *New Dimension in Solvent Formulation, Elvax Vinyl Resins,* DuPont Publication (1964)

(2)     Reference 49

Table 2. *Parameters Affecting Capsular Wall Permeability*

| POLYMERIC WALL MATERIAL | FOR LOWER PERMEABILITY |
|---|---|
| PARAMETERS (1) | |
| Density | Increase |
| Crystallinity | Increase |
| Orientation | Increase |
| Crosslinking | Increase |
| Plasticizer Level | Decrease |
| Fillers | (Increase) Conditional |
| Solvents Used in Film Preparation | Use Good Solvents Versus Poor |
| Solubility Parameter (2) | On the Opposite Side of SP Scale From Core Material |
| | |
| CAPSULAR PARAMETERS | |
| Size | Increase |
| Wall Thickness | Increase |
| Configuration | As Spherical As Possible |
| Conformity | As Regular As Possible |
| Post Treatments | Utilize |
| (Crosslinking, Sintering) | |
| Multiple Coatings | Utilize |
| ENVIRONMENTAL PARAMETERS | |
| Temperature, Storage | Decrease |
| Partial Pressure Differential | Decrease |
| (Inside and Outside of Capsule Wall) | |

(1) Reference (50)

(2) Reference (49)

Another investigator, Dr. Normal Li, ESSO Corporation, even
questioned the need for solic walls.  He devised a transient
capsular system composed of liquid interfaces to successfully
separate hydrocarbon mixtures (88).

Permeability

In all of this early work the key words were containment,
protection, and controlled release.  Release was effected either
by application of heat, pressure or solvent dissolution of the
capsular wall.  The rate of loss of encapsulated liquids is
dependent on:  1) the volatility of the liquid, 2) its solubility
in the capsule wall polymer, and 3) its diffusion through the
capsular wall.  The rate of loss one might expect from a typical
core material such as water is shown in Figure 6.

While the absolute value of 1/2-life also depends on the
pressure gradient factors between the interior and exterior of
the capsular wall, the effect of capsule size and capsule wall
thickness on core 1/2-life is clearly evident.  Figure 7 shows
the effect of capsular wall material choice on core 1/2-life.
Hydrophobic films such as polytriflorochloroethylene have much
lower water permeation than either nitrocellulose or cellulose
acetate (73-75).

Applications

The choice of polymer wall material is highly dependent on
the core material utilized.  Generally, polymeric materials at
the opposite end of the solubility parameter scale (74) from the
core material offer the most efficient containment.  This opposite effect is illustrated in Table 1, by listing the solubility
parameter of some common solvents and resins in opposing order.
Thus, to contain n-pentane, (a low solubility parameter material),
a hydrophilic polymer having a high solubility parameter, such as
polyvinyl alcohol or nylon, might be chosen.  Other parameters
affecting capsule wall permeability are listed in Table 2.

Figure 8 correlates the encapsulation process with the
capsule size ranges produced.  For instance, if a capsular product
between 50 and 100 microns is desired, one of the processes falling in that designated area would be chosen.

Conclusion

A diverse and practical science has emerged from the embryo
dreams of a young chemist in the 30's.  One might ask where do we
go from here.  Those in the field now know more about the

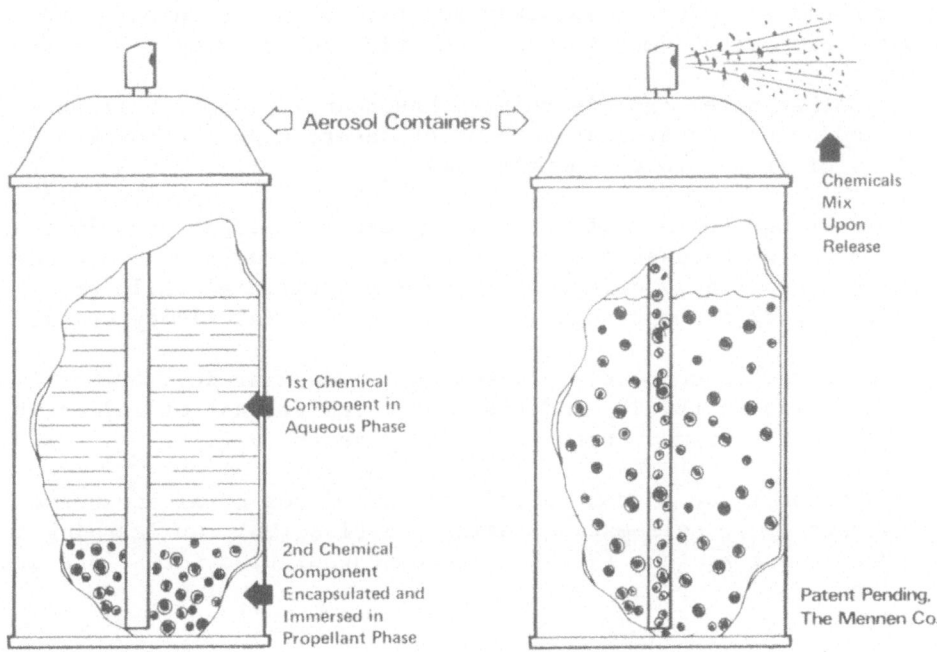

*Figure 10. Pressurized storage and depressurized release of microcapsules as a novel means of storage and instant activation of two-component chemical systems.*

capabilities and the practical limitations of microencapsulation. The science has become more exacting, but there is still room for other imaginative dreamers willing to put their ideas to work.

Novel methods of capsule release are still being discovered. One, utilizing pressure rupture, is shown in Figure 10. The capsules containing one reactant are stored in the propellant phase, while the second reactant is in the aqueous phase. Upon release from the pressurized container, the capsules rupture, releasing their chemical which immediately reacts. Products based on this process are being aimed for the cosmetic and adhesive fields (93).

Another novel capsule release has been employed in freeze-thaw indicators, useful as a means of determining the thermal history of frozen food products (94).

Pressing problems of our era suggest microcapsular solution. In bioscience, thousands of lives could be saved if we could only prepare biologically compatible capsular artificial cells or utilize capsular components in compact artificial kidney units.

Research is currently proceeding in capsular delivery of poison antidotes (89,90) and the controlled release of medications in the blood stream or through living tissues (91,92).

Whether it be in controlled release of potential environmental pollutants (95), self-extinguishing plastics (96), or learning how to control our weather (97,98), microencapsulation scientists are involved.

## ACKNOWLEDGEMENTS

The author wishes to thank Mr. Dan J. Kieffer, Mr. Dennis Orosz, and Mrs. Irma Brown for their assistance during the preparation of this article, and the many scientists in this field that provided specific historical information.

## REVIEW ARTICLES

I Harvard Business School, "Report on Microencapsulation" Management Reports, (1963).

II Flinn, J. E., and H. Nack, "What is Happening to Microencapsulation," Chem. Eng. p. 171 (Dec. 4, 1967).

III Herbig, J. E., Encyclopedia of Polymer Technology (1968).

IV Sirine, G., Microencapsulation, A Technique for Limitless Products, Food Products Development, (April-May 1968).

V Nack, H., Microencapsulation, Techniques, Applications and Problems, J. Soc. Cosmet, Chem., *21,* 85 (Feb. 4, 1970).

VI Luzzi, L. A., Microencapsulation, J. Phar. Sci., 1367 (1970).

VII Bakan, J., J. Anderson, Microencapsulation, *Industrial Pharmacology,* Lea & Febiger, (1970).

VIII Balassa, L. A., G. O. Fanger, Microencapsulation in the Food Industry, C.R.C. Critical Reviews, *2,* p. 245, (July 1971).

IX Chang, T. M. S., *Artificial Cells,* C. Thomas, (1972).

X McKernen, Flavour Industry, (December 1972 — January 1973).

XI Gutcho, M., *Capsule Technology and Microencapsulation,* Noyes Data Corp. (1972).

## REFERENCES

1   Sussman, A. H. Halvorson, *Spores, Their Dormancy and Germination* pp. 40-51, Harper & Row (1966).
2   Ibid. pp. 40-41
3   Rogers, H. J., H. R. Perkins, *Cell Walls and Membranes,* p. 372, E. & F.N. Spon Ltd. (1968).
4   Bungenburg de Jong, H. G., Proc., Acad. Sci. Amsterdam *41,* p. 646, (1938).
5   Bungenburg de Jong, H. G., Kass, Biochem. Zeit., *232,* p. 338, (1931).
6   Green, B. K., U.S. Reissue 24,899, (November 29, 1960).
7   Green, B. K., L. Schleicher, U.S. 2,800,457 and U.S. 2,800,458 (July 23, 1957).
8   Bakan, J. A., U.S. 3,436,355 (April 1, 1969).
9   Brynko, C., J. A. Scarpelli, U.S. 3,190,837 (June 22, 1965).
10  Yurkowitz, I. L., U.S. 3,533,958 (October 13, 1970).
11  Brynko C., J. A. Bakan, R. E. Miller, J. A. Scarpelli, U.S. 3,341,466 (September 12, 1967).

12   Jensen, E. H., U.S. 3,265,630 (August 9, 1966).

13   Brynko, C., J. A. Bakan, U.S. 3,401,123 (September 10, 1968).

14   Brynko, C., G. M. Olderman, U.S. 3,516,943 (June 23, 1970).

15   Striley, D. J., J. E. Williams, U.S. 3,520,821 (July 21, 1970).

16   Dobry, A., F. Boyer-Kawenoki, "Phase Separation in Polymer Solution," J. Poly. Sci., p. 90, (January 1947).

17   Powell, T. C., M. E. Steinle, R. A. Yoncoskie, U.S. 3,415,758 (December 10, 1965).

18   Miller, R. E., J. L. Anderson, U.S. 3,155,590 (November 3, 1964).

19   Rowe, H. L., U.S. 3,336,155 (August 15, 1967).

20   Fanger, G. O., R. E. Miller, R. G. McNiff, U.S. 3,531,418 (September 29, 1970).

21   Anderson, J. L., G. L. Gardner, N. H. Yoshida, U.S. 3,341,416 (September 12, 1967).

22   Gardner, G. L., *Manufacturing Encapsulated Products,* Chem. Engr. Prog., *62,* (4) pp. 87-91, (1966).

23   *The Use of Sustained Release Aspirin in Preparation and Management of Rheumatoid Arthritis,* J. of Clincal Phar. (March-April, 1967).

24   *Transient Surface Temperature Response of Liquid Crystals Cells,* Int. Liquid Crystal Conf. (August 1972).

25   *Development of Multipurpose Capsular Adhesives,* Picatinny Arsenal, U.S. Gov. Report No. DAAA-21-68c-0581.

26   Reyes, Z., U.S. 3,173,878 (March 16, 1965) and U.S. 3,405,070 (October 8, 1968).

27   Vassiliades, A. E., U.S. 3,418,656 and U.S. 3,418,250 (December 24, 1968).

28   Matson, G. W., U.S. 3,516,846 (June 23, 1970).

29   Baxter, G., U.S. 3,578,605 (May 11, 1971).

30   Taylor, H. F., U.S. 2,183,053 (1939) and U.S. 2,218,592 (1940).

31   Koff, A., P. F. Widmer, U.S. 3,143,475 (January 23, 1961).

32   Balassa, L., U.S. 3,495,988 (February 17, 1970).

33   Pasin, J. Z., U.S. 3,664,963 (May 23, 1972).

34   Ohtaki, S., U.S. 3,056,728 (October 14, 1958).

35   Klaui, H. M., W. Hausheer, G. Muschki, from I.E.F.N., *9, Fat Soluble Vitamins,* Edited by R. A. Morton, Pergamon Press Oxford (1970).

36   Private Communication, Polaks Frutal Works, Middletown, New York.

37   Schock, T. J., C. A. Spencer, U.S. 2,876,160 (March 3, 1959).

38   Wurzburg, O., W. Herbst, U.S. 3,091,567 (February 17, 1961).

39   Evans R., W. Herbst, U.S. 3,159,585 (April 12, 1961).

40   Marotta, N. G., et al, U.S. 3,455,838 (July 15, 1969).

41   Grevenstuk, A. B., F. Hougesteger, U.S. 3,202,731 (August 24, 1965).

42   Macaulay, N., U.S. 3,016,308 (January 9, 1962).

43   Miles, J. M., B. Mitzner, J. Brenner, E. Polak, "Encapsulated Perfumes in Aerosol Products," J. Soc. Cosmet, Chem., *22,* pp. 655-666 (September 17, 1971).

44   Sachsel, G. F., H. Nack, U.S. 3,202,533 (August 24, 1965).

45   Nack, H., U.S. 3,035,338 (May 29, 1962) and U.S. 3,382,093 (May 7, 1968).

46   Grass, G. M., M. J. Robinson, U.S. 3,237,596 (September 1961).

47   Powell, C. F., J. H. Oxley, and J. M. Blocker, Jr., Editors *Vapor Deposition,* John Wiley & Sons (1966).

48   Goldberger, W. M., C. J. Baroch, U.S. 3,247,014 (April 19, 1966).

49   Baer, C. A., U.S. 2,846,971.

50   Wurster, D. E., U.S. 2,648,609 (August 1953), U.S. 2,799,241 (July 1957), U.S. 3,089,824 (May 1963), U.S. 3,117,027 (January 1964), U.S. 3,196,827 (July 1965), U.S. 3,207,824 (April 1965), U.S. 3,241,520 (March 1966), U.S. 3,253,944 (May 1966).

51   Coletta, V., H. Rubin, *Wurster Coated Aspirin I,* J. Phar. Sci. Vol. 53, No. 8 (August 1964).

52    Wood, J., J. Syarbo, *Wurster Coated Aspirin II*, J. Phar. Sci. Vol 53, No. 8 (August 1964).

53    Schreiber, K., L. J. LaCroix, Can. J. Plant Sci., Vol. 47 (1967).

54    Somerville, G. R., U.S. 3,015,128 (January 2, 1962), U.S. 3,310,612 (March 21, 1967), and U.S. 3,389,194 (1968).

55    Langer, G., G. Yamate, *Encapsulation of Liquid and Solid Particles to Form Dry Powders*, J. Coll & Interface Sci., *29,* No. 3 (March 1969).

56    Berger, B., C. Miller, G. Langer, U.S. 3,208,951 (September 28, 1965).

57    Langer, G., G. Yamate, U.S. 3,159,874 (December 8, 1964).

58    Shultz, E., U.S. 2,857,281 (October 21, 1958).

59    Cardarelli, N. F., Rubber World, 166, p. 27 (August 1972).

60    Cardarelli, N. F., U.S. 3,417,181 (December 17, 1968), U.S. 3,590,119 (June 29, 1971), and U.S. 3,639,583 (February 1, 1973).

61    Rindt, D. R., G. M. Blouin, J. G. Getsinger, *Sulfur Coating on Nitrogen Fertilizer to Reduce Dissolution Rate*, J. A. gr. Food Chem., Vol. 16, No. 5 (September-October 1968).

62    Baymiller, J. W., W. J. Bohrn, and W. A. Moggio, U.S. 3,293,695 (December 27, 1966).

63    Arens, R. P., N. P. Swenny, U.S. 3,423,489 (January 21, 1969).

64    Raley, C. F., W. J. Burkett, Jr., and J. S. Swearinger, U.S. 2,766,478 (Ocotber 16, 1956).

65    Bentov, I., and R. M. Jolkovski, U.S. 3,167,602 (January 26, 1965).

66    Herman, D. F., U. Kruse, J. J. Brancato, *Polyethylene Encapsulated Cellulose*, J. Poly. Sci. Part C. No. 11, pp. 75-95 (1965).

67    Herman, D. F., U. Kruse, U.S. 3,297,466 (January 10, 1967).

68    Gorham, W. F., U.S. 3,288,728 (February 18, 1966) and U.S. 3,342,754 (February 18, 1966).

69    Gorham, W. F., H. L. Willard, U.S. 3,300,332 (February 7, 1966).

70    Gorham, W. F., Sci., *4,* 3027 (1966).

71    Robbins, R. C., U.S. 3,219,476 (November 23, 1965).

72    Chemical Week, p. 76, (February 11, 1967).

73    Brandrup, J., E. H. Immergut, *Polymer Handbook,* V-13, V-21, Interscience Publishers (1967).

74    Hildebrand, J. H., R. L. Scott, "The Solubility of Nonelectrolytes," 3rd ed., Reinhold, New York (1950).

75    Briston, J. H., *Permeability of Plastic, The Flavor Industry,* pp. 779-783 (November 1970).

76    Morgan, P. W., S. L. Kuclek, Interfacial Polymerization, J. Poly. Sci., *40,* 299 (1959).

77    Vandegaer, J. E., F. G. Meyer, U.S. 3,464,926 (September 2, 1969).

78    Doyle, A. W., R. M. Jolkovski, A. C. Laws, U.S. 3,160,686 (December 8, 1964).

79    Jolkovski, R. M., A. C. Laws, D. H. Powers, U.S. 3,270,100 (August 30, 1966).

80    Santo, J. E., J. E. Vandegaer, U.S. 3,492,380 (January 27, 1970).

81    Levine, S. N., W. C. La Course, *Materials & Design Considerations for a Compact Artificial Kidney,* J. Biomed. Met. Res., *1,* 275 (67).

82    Sparks, R. F., R. M. Salamine, P. M. Meier, M. H. Litt, O. Lindan, *Removal of Waste Metabolites in Uremia by Microcapsular Reactants,* Trans. Am. Soc. Art. Inter. Organs, *15,* 353, (1969).

83    Chang, T. M. S., Semi Permeable Microcapsules, Sci, *146,* 524, (1964).

84    Chang, T. M. S., *Artificial Cells,* Chapt. 9, Thomas (1972).

85    Chang, T. M. S., U.S. 3,522,346 (July 28, 1970).

86    Shigeri, Y., T. Kondo, et al., *Studies on Microcapsules: Variation in Microcapsule Size,* Can. J. Chem., *48,* 2047 (70).

87    Chang, T. M. S., *Artificial Cells,* Chapt. 5, Thomas (1972).

88    Li, N., *Separating Hydrocarbons with Liquid Membranes,* U.S. 3,410,794 (1966) and U.S. 3,410,078 (1966).

89    Done, A. K., *Treatment of Salicylate Poisoning,* Mod. Treatment, *4,* p. 648 (1967).

90    Chang, T. M. S., *Artificial Cells,* pp. 141, 145, Thomas (1972).

91    *New Delivery Systems May Recast Drug Therapy,* C. & E. News (September 6, 1971).

92    Alza Corporation, U.S. 3,598,122 and U.S. 3,598,123.

93    Private Communication, The Mennen Company, Morristown, New Jersey.

94    Food Processing, p. 32 (October 1972) and Artech Corporation, Private Communication, Falls Church, Virginia.

95    *Microcapsular Controlled Usage of Agriculture Adjuvants,* Depts. of Biology, Environment & Chem. Newsletter, Battelle Columbus Labs, Issue 29, (November 1972-January 1973).

96    Praetzel, H. E., H. Jenkner, U.S. 3,660,321 (May 2, 1972).

97    *Cloud Seeding of Microencapsulated Materials,* U.S. Gov. Phbl. A.S.C.R.L. -71-0151 (February 1971).

98    Nelson, L. D., B. A. Silverman, U.S. 3,659,785 (May 2, 1972).

# ENCAPSULATION BY COACERVATION

Jan E. Vandegaer*

Before going into a detailed description of this method of encapsulation it will be necessary to describe hydrophilic colloids and the ways in which they undergo coacervation.

## HYDROPHILIC COLLOIDS

Hydrophilic colloids are large molecules which are dispersible or soluble in water or aqueous solutions. They can be of natural origin or can be synthesized. Examples of natural hydrophilic colloids are the following: Gelatin, alginates, albumin, casein, agar-agar, gum arabic, pectins and starch. Some of these colloidal materials are not obtained directly from nature, but have undergone some modification. One of them is carboxymethylcellulose which is the natural material cellulose which has undergone a chemical reaction. As a matter of fact it is quite difficult to remove any colloidal material from its natural environment without modifying it in the process. Other hydrophilic colloids are synthesized outright, such as polyacrylic acid, polyacrylamide, etc.

The gelatin molecule is made up of amino acids joined together by peptide linkages in a long molecular chain. There are 18 different $\alpha$-amino acids in gelatin, each occuring at its own proportion and sequence in the large molecules. The linkages involving the carboxylic groups and the alpha-amino groups form the backbone of the molecule. The rest of each amino acid is known as side-chain. These side-chains can contain basic amino or guanidine groups or acidic carboxyl groups. For instance, lysine

*Address correspondence c/o Plenum Publishing Corporation, 227 W. 17th St., New York, N. Y. 10011.

carries an extra amino group, arginine carries a guanidine group, whereas aspartic acid and glutamic acid carry extra carboxylic groups.

Gum arabic on the other hand has the following composition (1):

            30.3% of L-Arabinose
            11.4% of L-Rhamnose
            36.8% of D-Galactose
            13.8% of D-Glucuronic acid

Gum Arabic does not contain any basic groups and therefore never carries a positive charge. The glucuronic acid ionizes in neutral and basic medium to a negatively charged anion.

Hydrophilic colloids which are of interest for coacervation are present in water in the form of loosely kinked coils as depicted in Figure 1.

These colloids have several ionizable groups along their chain which exchange protons and other ions with the surrounding aqueous medium, and thereby acquire charges. For instance, a

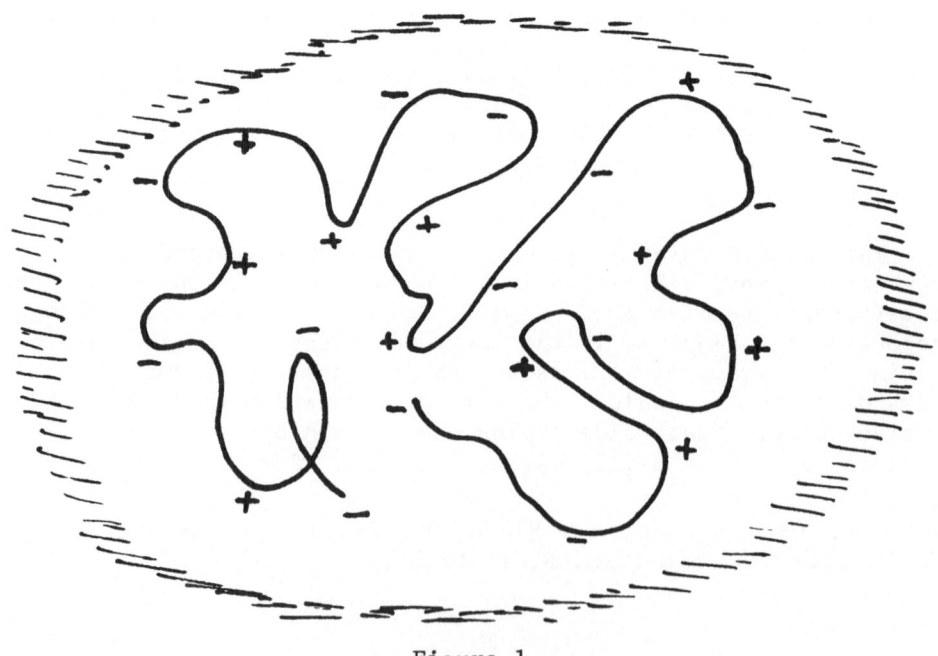

Figure 1

carboxylic acid group on gum arabic in water of neutral pH will be
ionized to the carboxylate ion and thereby give the chain a negative charge. On the other hand an amine group on gelatin will at
neutral pH attract a proton from the surrounding aqueous medium
and form a positively charged $NH_3^+$-group. These charges along the
macromolecular chain in solution hold the polar water molecules
with varying strengths depending on how far the water molecules
are from the chain. Thus every colloid macromolecule in solution
more or less controls an envelope of water. It is this partially
bound water which helps keep the macromolecule in solution.
Therefore, the solubility or the dispersibility of a colloid is
very much a function of its charge.

This charge is in turn a function of the pH of the aqueous
medium. For instance, the carboxylic acid groups which are
ionized into carboxylate ions at neutral or basic pH will lose
their negative charge at a more acid pH. Conversely the amino
groups which carry a positive charge at neutral and acid pH will
return to their simple amino or $-NH_2$ configuration at basic pH.
The fact that the charge of a hydrophilic colloid is often a function of pH can be demonstrated quite readily by means of the
Burton tube as shown in Fig. 2.

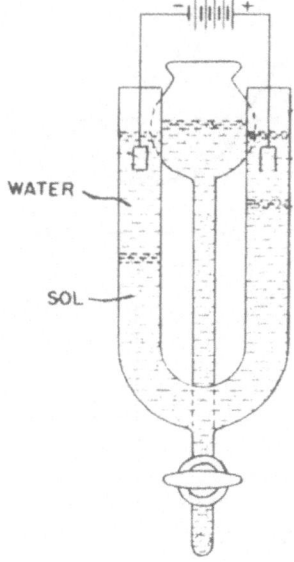

WATER

SOL

Figure 2

A colloidal solution or sol, in equilibrium with a buffer
solution at a certain pH, is placed in a U tube. Buffer solution
is added to both legs of the U tube. Two electrodes, one in each
leg, are inserted in the buffer solution. When a potential difference is applied between the electrodes, the colloid will move to
one or the other electrode. If the colloid carries a net positive
charge it will move to the negative electrode. If it has a net
negative charge it will move to the positive electrode. The rate
of movement or electrophorectic mobility of a colloid at constant
electrode potential is a measure of the net colloidal charge. The
relationship between colloid charge and pH can be determined
experimentally by using different buffer solutions and thus
depicted graphically as in Figure 3.

A colloid with a net positive charge can be called a colloid
cation. Similarly, a colloid with a net negative charge can be
called a colloid anion.

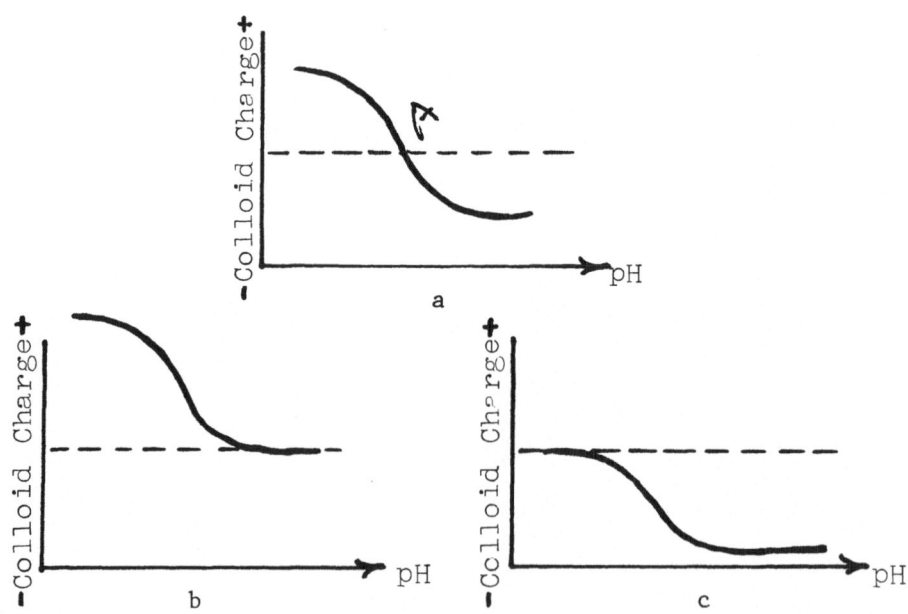

Figure 3

Fig. 3a is representative of a hydrophilic colloid which is amphoteric in nature such as gelatin.  The net positive charge at low pH results from protonated amino groups while the negative charge at high pH is due to carboxylate anions.  A colloid containing only basic groups (e.g. a polyamine) would carry no negative charge and would have a curve as in 3b.  On the other hand, a colloid such as gum arabic which has only acid groups would never carry a positive charge and would give a relationship as in 3c.

The point A in Fig. 3a is called the isoionic point (I) or the isoionic pH value.  This simply represents the point at which the net colloid charge is zero.

In practice the isoelectric point (IEP) is more commonly used.  It differs slightly from the isoionic point in that it takes into account not only the charges on the macromolecule proper, but also the charges due to small salt ions that may be absorbed from the solution and migrate with the colloid.

It is possible to change the charge pattern of an hydrophilic colloid as shown in Fig. 4.

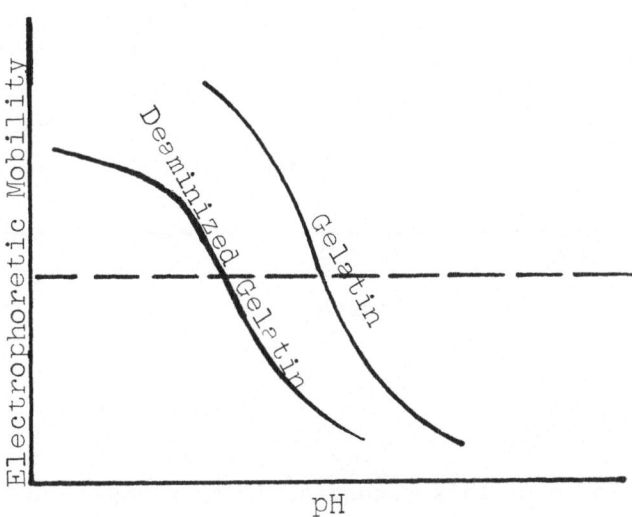

Figure 4

The two curves shown represent one of normal gelatin and one of gelatin which has had some of its amino groups removed by a de-amination reaction. On the ordinate axis the electrophoretic mobility of the colloid is plotted as a function of the pH of the aqueous medium. Since all or a large portion of the amino groups have been eliminated in the deaminized gelatin, the total charge has become less positive and therefore the isoelectric point is shifted to a lower pH value.

If we now compare two hydrophilic colloids with different isoelectric points as shown in Fig. 5, one can readily see that in the pH region between the two isoelectric points A&B, the colloids will have opposite charges. The colloid with isoelectric point B will have a positive charge whereas the colloid with iso-electric point A will have a negative charge.

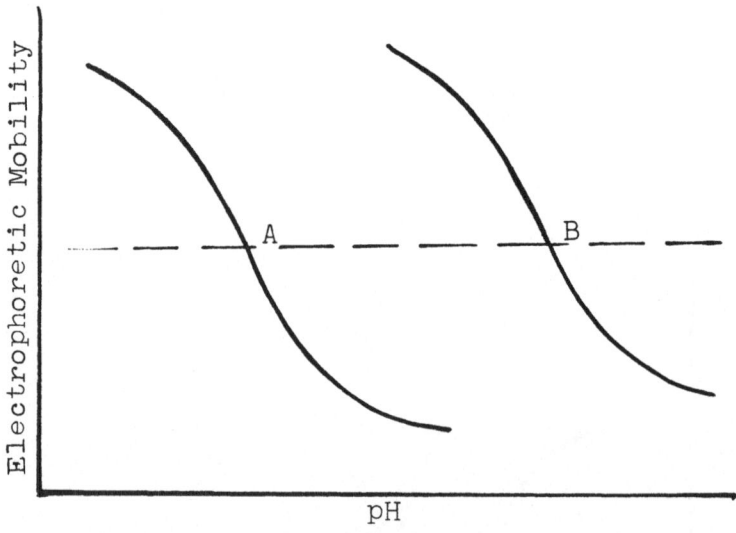

Figure 5

Characteristic of this situation is an example involving gum arabic and gelatin. In the region of neutral pH (6-8), gelatin carries a net positive charge while gum arabic is negative. See Fig. 6.

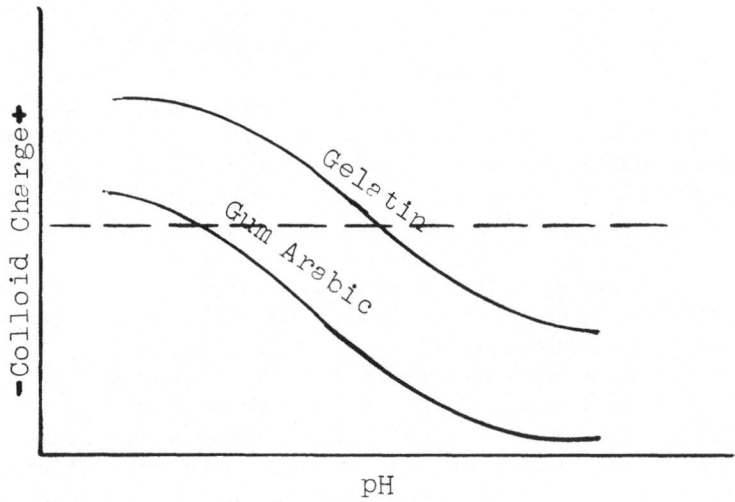

Figure 6

## COACERVATION

About forty years ago, two Dutch scientists suggested for the first time the name of coacervation to describe the phenomenon of phase separation in colloidal systems. The phenomenon of phase separation into colloid-rich and a colloid-poor layers had already been observed before, but these authors for the first time described it in a systematic way. They realized that this phase separation they called "coacervation" was very closely related to the precipitation or flocculation of the colloidal material from solution and that coacervation was merely a step taking place just before precipitation from solution.

Since the term "partial miscibility" already had a well defined meaning, namely - the separation of one phase into two coexisting phases, it appeared desirable not to use the same term for the formation of two liquid layers in hydrophilic colloids. Consequently, they introduced the term "coacervation" from the Latin "acervus" meaning agregation, and the prefix "co" to signify the preceeding union of the colloidal particles. Coacervates are colloid-rich solutions.

The unique property of coacervation systems is the fact that the solvent components of the two phases are the same. This is the basic distinguishing characteristic of a coacervate as

compared to two-phase systems involving two immiscible liquids.
Thus, a colloidal solute particle migrating across the interphase
of a two-phase coacervate system finds itself in essentially the
same environment on either side of the interphase. From the view-
point of composition, the difference between two phases is a
difference in concentration of solute species.

There are essentially two methods of coacervation, simple and
complex. The simple method involves the removal of the aqueous
solvation layer around the hydrophilic colloids, whereas the
complex method of coacervation has to do with the charges on the
colloid and their neutralization. Simple coacervation is caused
by the removal of the associated water layer from around the
dissolved colloid chain. This can be accomplished by the addition
of chemical compounds with great affinity for water such as salts
or alcohols. Such compounds will compete with the colloid for the
associated water molecules. When the colloid chain loses enough
of its water molecules it coacervates with other colloid chains.
This occurs because the colloid chains are no longer isolated from
each other. Once these now less hydrophilic chains touch they
tend to associate and intertwine thus penetrating each other's
domain.

Water removal from the colloid coil by the addition of
alcohol is illustrated in Fig. 7 by a ternary phase diagram.

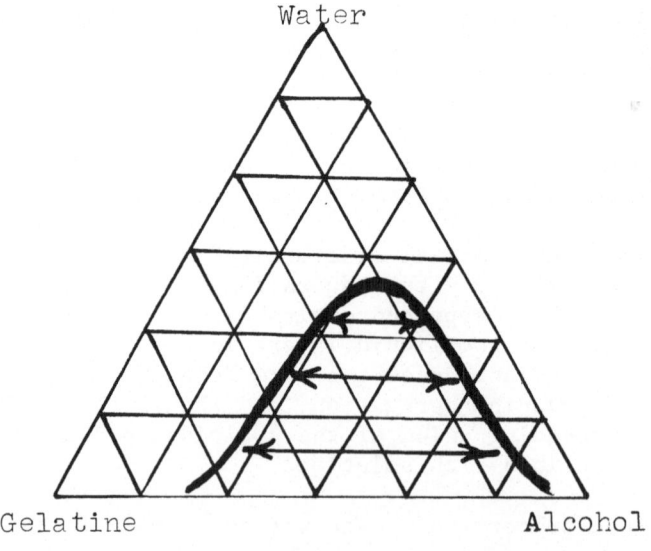

Figure 7

The zone of immiscibility of coacervation is below the curve
and close to the higher alcohol concentration.  The tielines in
the diagram indicate that the water and alcohol solution left in
in the coacervate must be less concentrated in alcohol than the
solution with which the coacervate is in equilibrium.  Fig. 8 is
an example of coacervation brought about by the addition of a salt
solution - namely a 20% ammonium sulphate solution.  The example
is taken from U. S. Patent 2,800,458 issued to B. Green.

The region to the right of line 33 is the coacervate region
of the mixture.  The right-hand side of the immiscibility region
is not drawn on this diagram.

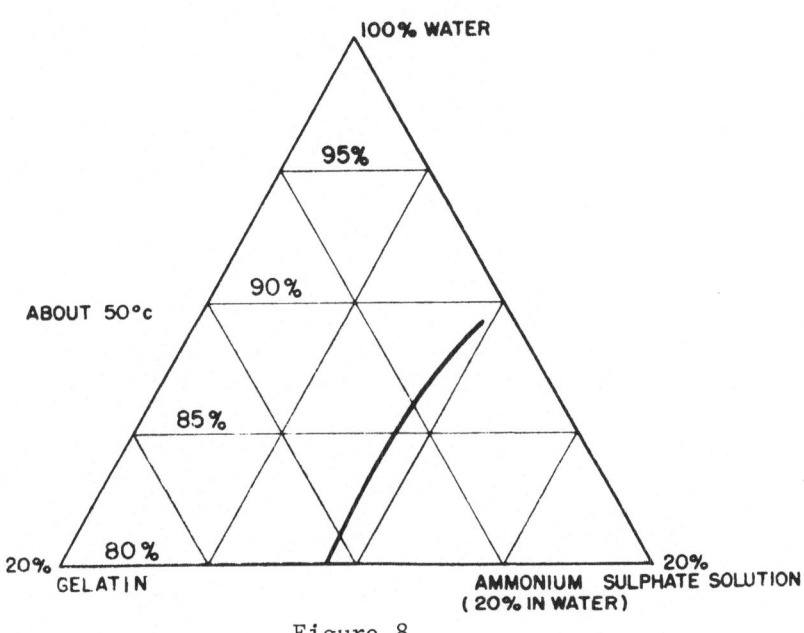

Figure 8

Complex coacervation on the other hand involves the neutralization of the charges on the colloid.  This is accomplished by
mixing two colloids together which carry opposite charges.  From
the previous part of this chapter it can be gathered that a
combination of gelatin and gum arabic at neutral pH will fulfill
this condition.  For instance, at that pH gelatin carries a net
positive charge because of protonation of basic groups, whereas
gum arabic carries a negative charge because of the ionization of
the glucuronic acid groups.  These two colloids attract each other
and they separate into a distinct liquid phase called "the
coacervate".

The two phases are essentially the same except that in the
coacervate the colloid concentration is much higher than in the
other phase.  The following <u>ternary</u> phase diagram illustrates the
coacervation occurring at fairly high dilution in water - the area
in which this happens is located at the top of the triangle (2).

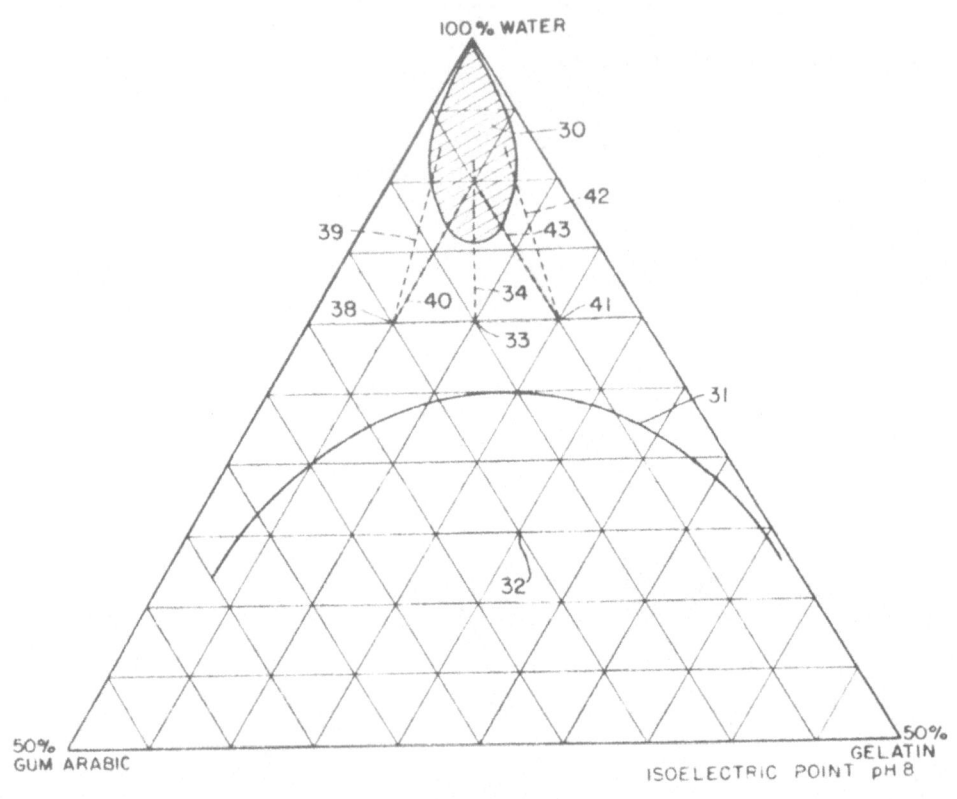

Figure 9

H. R. Kruyt in the second volume of Colloid Science published
by Elsevier in 1949 describes complex coacervation as follows
(page 339).  "If one adds a little HCl to a warm mixture of dilute
gelatin and gum arabic salts, complex coacervation first takes
place at a certain pH value below 4.8, the isoelectric point of
the gelatin used, the liquid becomes turbid and the presence of
coacervate drops can be readily detected by means of a microscope.

If one adds some sodium hydroxide to a pH above 4.8, the co-acervation disappears, again to recur after acidification" This obviously happens because above 4.8 both colloids are negatively charged. "This appearance and disappearance of coacervation can be repeated a number of times. It can happen, however, that with an increasing number of repetitions of alternate additions of sodium hydroxide and HCl, the turbidity becomes steadily weaker and finally does not occur at all. This is explained by the formation of an increasing amount of sodium chloride. It is, in fact, characteristic of complex coacervation that it is hindered by indifferent salts at sufficiently high salt concentration or, if it already has a coacervate system, the coacervation is suppressed by the addition of an indifferent salt."

Since a positively charged colloid and a negatively charged colloid neutralize each other, it results in an overall reduction of the net charge, and the partial loss of solvation water of these colloidal species. This preceeds generally the precipitation of the two oppositely charged colloids from solution and may also be regarded as the cause of the phase separation in the complex coacervation system. However, while the reduction of the net charge is a necessary precondition of complex coacervation, it is frequently not enough to achieve it. A lowering of temperature often helps. In other words, the reduction of the overall charge on the colloidal particles must alter or modify the attraction between the colloids and the water to such an extent that the colloidal particles will tend to aggregate to form a distinct, continuous liquid phase rather than a flocculent or solid phase. This tendency to aggregate is attributable to long range Van der Waal's interaction of the colloids in solution when after loss of charge and water they have become more hydropholic in the aqueous medium.

In both "simple" and "complex" coacervation, two-solution phase formation begins with the colloidal species aggregating to form sub-microscopic cluster  These clusters coalesce to form microscopic droplets. Further coalescence produces microscopic droplets which tend to separate into a continuous phase.

## ENCAPSULATION

Now that coacervation of hydrophilic colloids has been explained, it should be easy to understand how the encapsulation procedure is performed.

Capsules are made by dispersion of oil in small droplets in the aqueous phase containing the hydrophilic colloid. If these oil droplets are properly dispersed and stabilized  if necessary, coacervation can be brought about and the capsules formed.

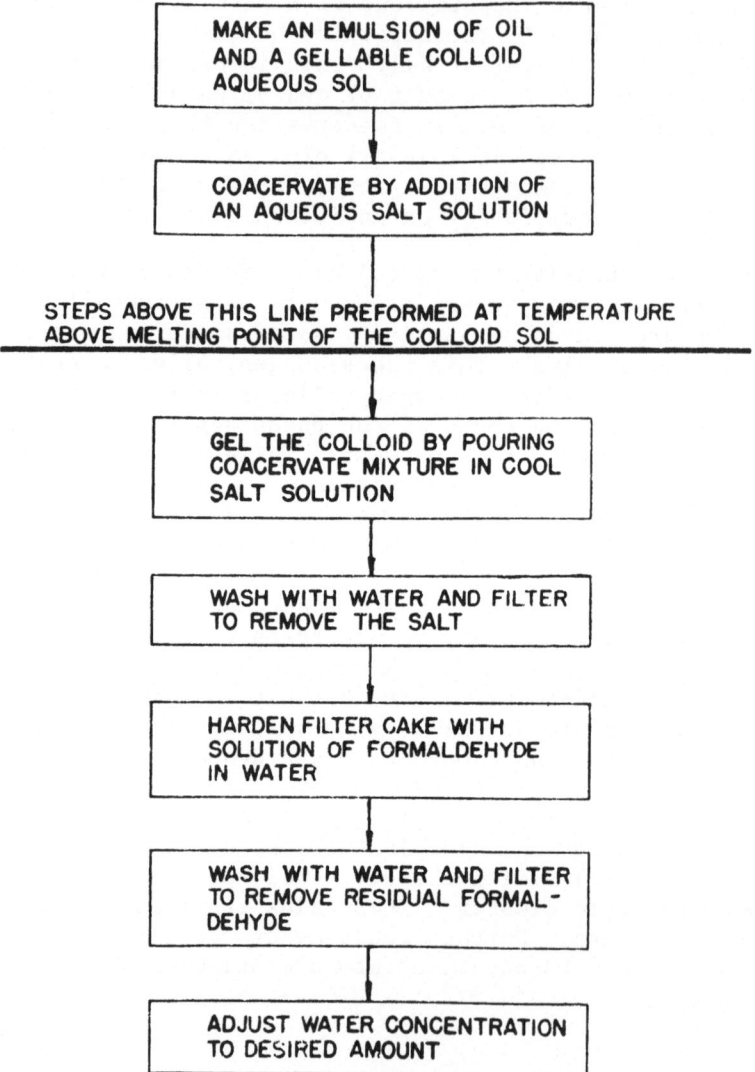

Figure 10

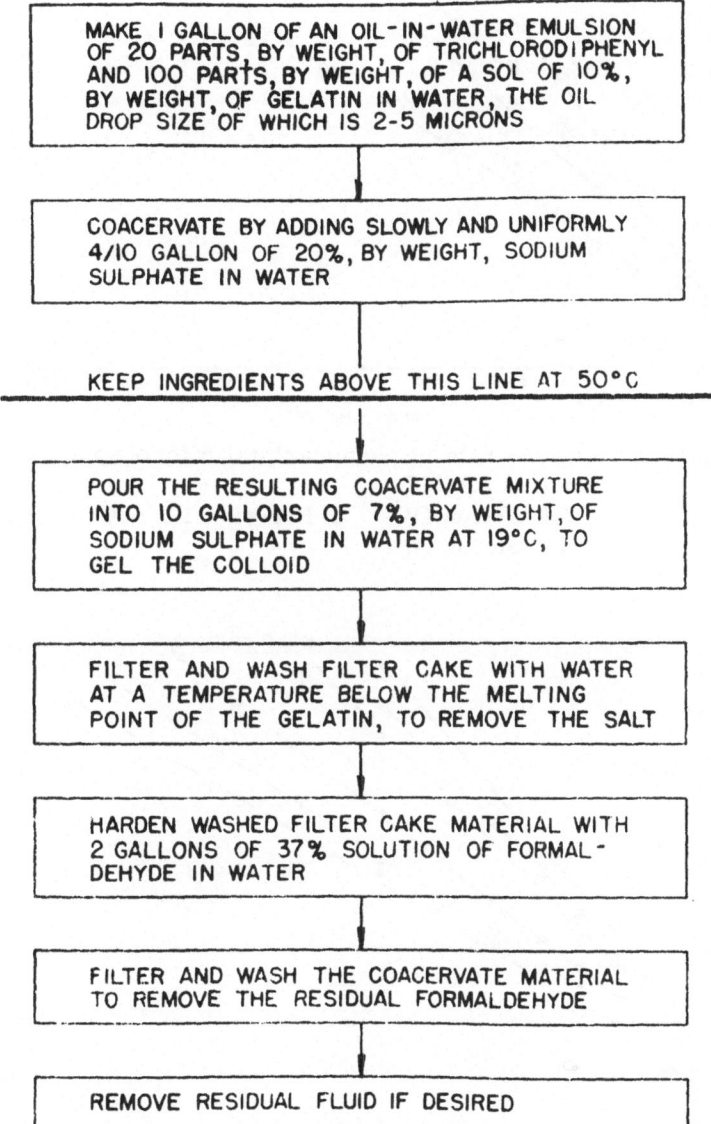

Figure 11

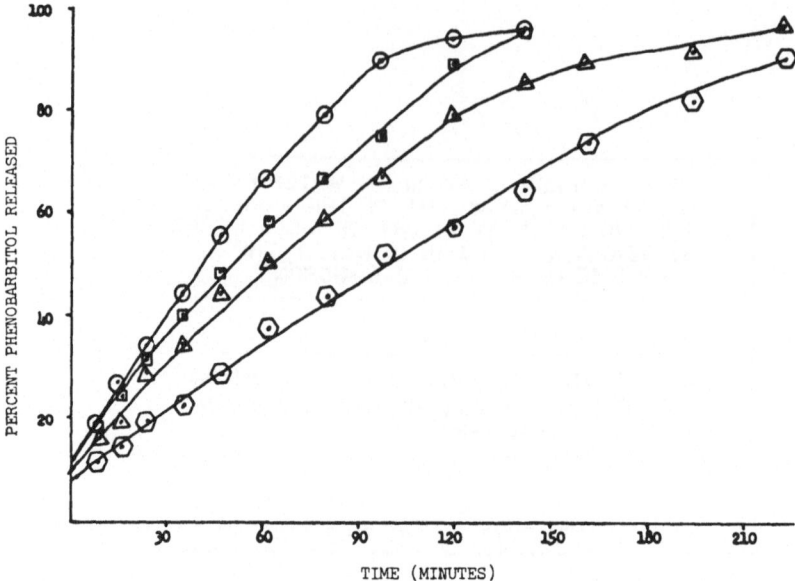

Figure 1.  Release rate of phenobarbital microcapsule pre-
           pared at pH 3.7.
               ⊙Fraction IV      ⊡ Fraction I      ▲ Fraction II
               ⊚ Fraction III

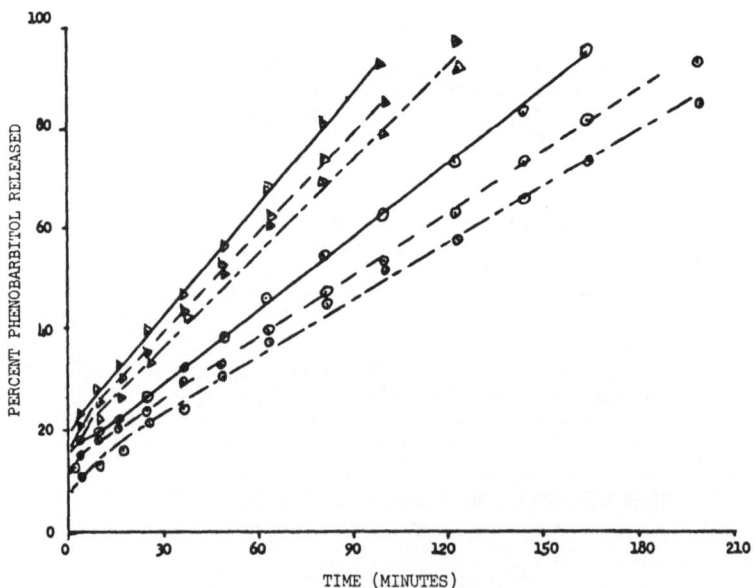

Figure 2.  Release rate of phenobarbital microcapsules as
           a function of pH of preparation
               △ Fraction I       O Fraction III
           ――――― pH 4.2   ― ― ― pH 3.2   ―・―・― pH 3.7

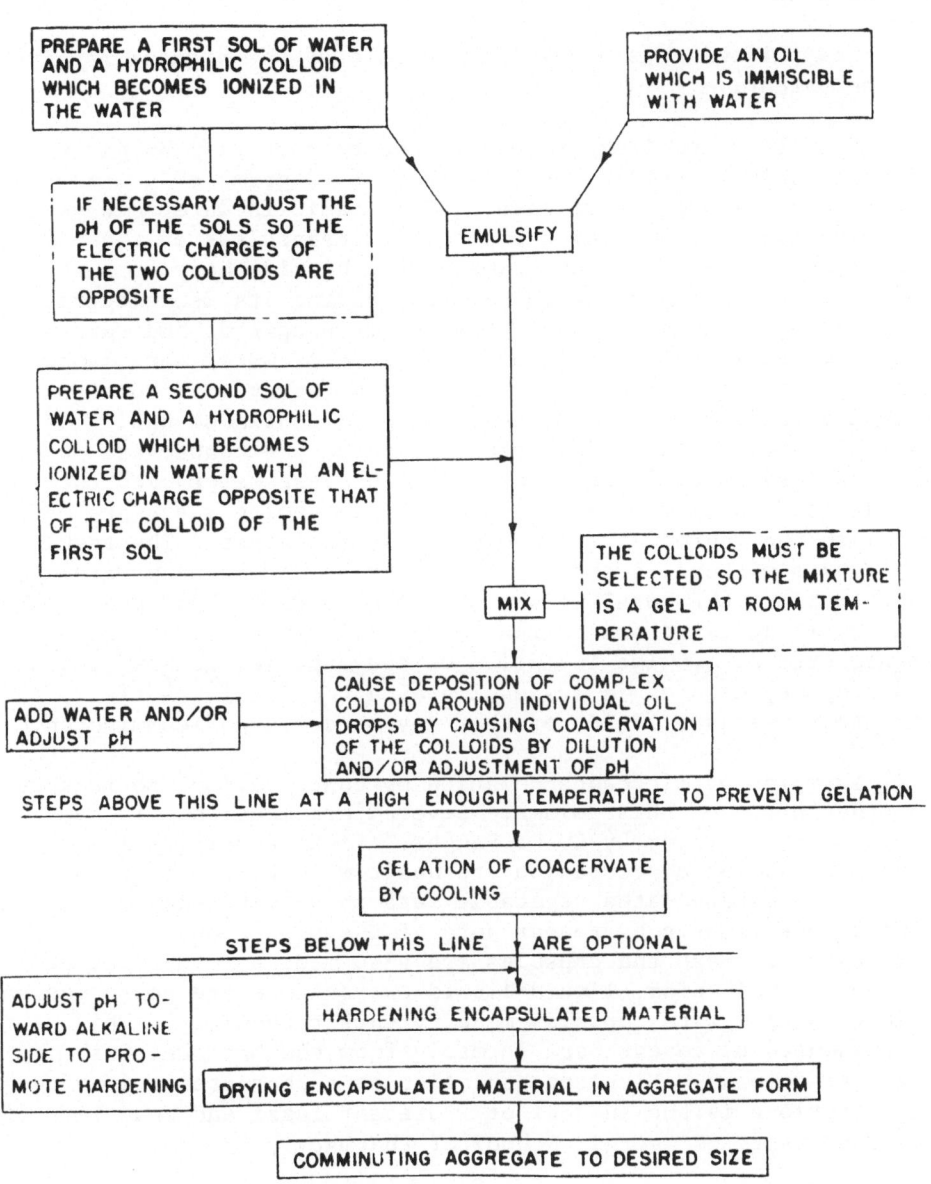

Figure 12

taken from Patent 2,800,457, illustrates the procedure in a
general way.  Here again the coacervation is performed at a certain
temperature, then later on the gellation of the coacervate is
brought about by cooling and, if necessary, hardening with
chemical additives.

The following is a specific example of the process as given
in the patent.

"First, a specific example of the process will be given, when
dilution only is used.  A sol is made of 20 grams of gum arabic
dissolved in 160 grams of water.  Gum arabic in water always forms
negative ions, it not being amphoteric, regardless of the pH.
Into this is emulsified 80 grams of trichloridiphenyl.  A second
sol of 20 grams of pork skin gelatin, having its iso-electric
point at pH 8, and 160 grams of water is prepared, and this second
sol is mixed with the emulsion.  A volume of water then is added
slowly to the mixture drop by drop, or by spray with constant
stirring until coacervation starts and is continued until the
particle size of the oil droplets on which the coacervate material
is deposited is as large as desired, the less water used the
smaller the particle size.  All of the foregoing steps are carried
out with the ingredients at 50 degrees centigrade.  The resulting
coacervate mixture is poured into water at $0^{\circ}$C, enough water being
used to bring the total weight of ingredients to 3960 grams.  The
mixture is agitated and thereafter is allowed to stand for an hour
at not over $25^{\circ}$C.  The formation of the capsules is now completed,
and they may be used in suspension as a coating for surfaces or
for other use as a fluid, or they may be dried and comminuted."

Examples of microencapsulation by coacervation are featured
in other parts of this volume.  Several are mentioned in the
introductory charter by G. O. Fanger.  Light sensitive microcapsules made by coacervation are dealt with by Professor S. Kubo.
The use of encapsulated vegetable fats in cattle feeds is the subject of one chapter by researchers of the Department of
Agriculture.  Here the capsules are also made by coacervation.  In
another contribution, liquid-liquid extractions are performed on
columns packed with capsules made by this technology.  This paper
is presented by researchers formerly from the National Cash
Register Company.  Microencapsulation as a characteristic of gelatin fractions is the subject of Professor Luzzi and coworkers of
the University of Georgia School of Pharmacy.

All the above examples illustrate the various ways in which
microcapsules made by coacervation can be used in the field.  Of
course, the largest application of all is the one that was the
major goal of inventor Barret Green and his coworkers when they
set out to make carbonless carbon paper which is illustrated in
the introductory chapter.

## REFERENCES

(1)  Butler, C. L. and Cretcher, L. H.   Journal of the American
     Chemical Society 52, 4509 (1930)

(2)  U.S. 2,800,457 B. K. Green et.al. (July 23, 1957)

# ENCAPSULATION OF SPHERICAL PARTICLES AS A

# CHARACTERISTIC OF GELATIN FRACTIONS

P. L. Madan, J. C. Price, L. A. Luzzi

Department of Pharmacy
University of Georgia
Athens, Georgia 30602

Both ethanol (1-4, 8, 9) and detergent-gelatin (4, 10) fractionation procedures have been reported in the literature. For this work, gelatin has been fractionated by using the coacervation process with acetone being used as coacervating agent.

In earlier literature (11-15), it has been shown that unfractionated gelatin was suitable as a part of complex coacervation encapsulation system.

Green and Schleicker (16-18), Jensen and Wagner (19), and Green (20) were early patentees to have used a gelatin-acacia system of complex coacervation to encapsulate various oils, some of which contained dissolved dyes. Luzzi and Gerraughty (13) encapsulated solid particles of colloidal sulfur, special flowers of sulfur, aspirin anhydride, acetophenetidin, barbituric acid, lycopodium spores, DDT, Pentobarbituric acid, and carbon black using a similar system of complex coacervation.

The process of microencapsulation has been used for a wide variety of applications. To name a few: solids, liquids or gases have been encapsulated to protect, separate, aid in storage and handling, and for sustained release of medicaments. From the pharmaceutical standpoint, microencapsulation has been used for taste masking, e. g., aspirin,

chlorpheniramine maleate, meprobromates (21, 22); for stabilization to oxidation, e.g., vitamin A palmitate (23); for reduction
of volatility as well as taste and odor masking, e.g., carbon
tetrachloride; and last but not the least, for sustained release,
e.g., d-amphetamine, aspirin, menthol, methyl salicylate-
camphor mixture (24, 25, 26).

That microencapsulation is finding increased use in
pharmaceuticals from both clinical and therapeutic aspects is
becoming more apparent. Undoubtedly the success of such a
procedure will depend on the wall thickness and/or toughness of
the encapsulating material. Unfortunately, the literature on
microencapsulation is not extensive and most of it comes from
company brochures or U.S. patents. A search of the literature
indicates that very few reports have been made on studies relevant to the wall thickness of microcapsules prepared by coacervation (12. 27, 28). Nixon et al (27) used the gelatin/sulfamera-
zine ratio as a measure of wall thickness in studying encapsulation of sulfamerazine by simple coacervation. Although complex
coacervation is one of the oldest methods known among the various methods that have been used for microencapsulation, only
two reports (11, 28) seem to have been made on the wall thickness
of microcapsules prepared by complex coacervation. Madan (11)
computed the wall thickness of microcapsules of spherical particles of stearyl alcohol made by complex coacervation based on
volume - surface area calculations for thin walled capsules.
Luu et al. (28) studied the diffusion and wall thickness of microcapsules containing a liquid organic base encapsulated by complex coacervation.

This investigation was therefore undertaken to fractionate
gelatin into various molecular weight size fractions, encapsulate
spherical particles of a solid material with the various gelatin
fractions via complex coacervation, collect the encapsulated
particles in the form of a free flowing powder, evaluate the wall
thickness of the microcapsules, study the release rate of the
encapsulated solid, and study the relationship between the wall
thickness and release rate of microcapsules prepared with each
of the gelatin fractions.

## Experimental

Materials: All materials used were of USP reagent or better
grade and except for the gelatin were used without further

purification.

Preparation of Internal Phase:  Reproducibility of the phase to be
encapsulated was insured by forming spherical particles of
phenobarbituric acid according to the method reported by Madan
et al. (12) for the preparation of stearyl alcohol.

Fractionation of Gelatin:  The method used for fractionation of
gelatin was based on the method of Pouradier and Venet (8) except that acetone was used as the fractionating agent.  A 5% dispersion of gelatin in water was prepared by first soaking Type A
Pigskin gelatin* in water for one hour at room temperature, and
then heating to 45-50$^{\circ}$, and swirling to effect a homogeneous
dispersion.  The pH of the dispersion was adjusted to 8.6 (the
pI of gelatin) and acetone, also at 45-50$^{\circ}$, slowly added, with
vigorous swirling, until cloudiness appeared.  The container was
stoppered and placed in a thermostatically controlled water-bath
at 37 $\pm$ 0.5$^{\circ}$.  The coacervate droplets producing the cloudiness
were allowed to form a coherent viscous layer.  The bulky
supernatant layer was then removed and retained for further
fractionation.

The coacervate layer was washed into teflon coated pans
and the solution was allowed to set to a gel and then dried in a
current of sterile filtered air.  Second, third, and fourth fractions were collected by continued addition of acetone.

Isoionic Point Determination:  The gelatin fractions were purified
by dialysis against distilled water at about 4$^{\circ}$.  The last three
washings were carried out with boiled, glass-distilled water to
remove traces of $CO_2$.

The Isoionic points were determined by measuring the pH
of the gelatin solution after all the salt had been removed by
dialysis.

Viscosity Measurements:  Two factors dictated the use of room
temperature for the determination of the viscosity of the gelatin
solutions:  (i) to avoid hydrolytic degradation, and (ii) convenience in density determination.

Potassium thiocyanate was used as the gelation-inhibiting
agent for the viscosity determinations.  It has been shown by
Kraemer (29) and a number of other investigators (8. 30, 31,

32-34) that gelatin is molecularly dispersed in 2M potassium
thiocyanate at room temperature.   Although Carpenter and
others (32-34) observed that 1 molal potassium thiocyanate
sufficed to prevent gelation down to 0.5°, the higher concentration of 2M was adopted to insure the maximum effect associated
with gelation prevention.

A simple U-tube Ostwald capillary viscometer was used
to determine the viscosities of gelatin solutions after the viscometer had been calibrated by measuring the flow time of distilled water and of potassium thiocyanate solution.   Density
determinations were done pycometrically.

Solutions were prepared containing 0.1%, 0.2%, 0.5%,
0.75%, and 1.0% gelatin in 2M potassium thiocyanate.   The
solutions were centrifuged for 30 minutes at a setting of 40 to
remove suspended matter.   The flow time through the viscometer of each centrifuged solution was determined accurately
to within 0.1 second with a stop watch.

The intrinsic viscosities of the unfractionated gelatin and
gelatin fractions were then found graphically by plotting reduced
viscosity as a function of concentration and extrapolating the
straight lines to zero concentration.

Encapsulation Procedure:   All work was conducted under identical experimental conditions.   Coacervation was carried out at
40° using a water bath maintained at 40 ± 1°.   In all experiments, gelatin and acacia solutions were prepared by dissolving,
separately, equal quantities of gelatin and acacia in 20 ml. of
distilled water.   These solutions were allowed to hydrate for at
least 12 hours before being used.

The method used for preparing the coacervate capsules
was based on the work of Luzzi and Gerraughty (13), except
that the phenobarbituric acid spheres were incorporated and the
collection procedure was adjusted.   For the work reported here,
the mixture from the coacervated encapsulation system was
filtered through a coarse filter paper and the coacervate was
resuspended in 100 ml. of 50% isopropanol.   Treatment with
isopropanol had a dehydrating and deflocculating effect.   The
mixture was again filtered using a coarse filter paper and then

air-dried at room temperature to yield a free flowing powder. The encapsulation process was followed microscopically.

This process of microencapsulation was repeated to prepare microcapsules using unfractionated gelatin and using the four collected gelatin fractions.

Effect of pH: Since complex coacervation is pH dependent, it was decided to study the wall thickness and release rate relationship of capsules made with gelatin fractions I and III as a function of pH of preparation of microcapsules. All variables were kept constant except that the pH of preparation was varied from 3.7 to 3.2 for one batch and 4.2 for the other batch.

Determination of Wall Thickness: The wall material was recovered from the encapsulated particles by extraction of phenobarbital with ethanol by the process reported by Madan (11).

In Vitro Dissolution Studies: Dissolution was followed by examining triplicate samples containing approximately 30 mg. of drug using the modified beaker method (35). The method consisted of 500-ml., three-necked round-bottom flask, with a 6-cm. hole cut in the center to accommodate the entrance of a 5-cm. propeller. A 300 ml. quantity of the dissolution medium (0.1N HCl), preheated to $37^{\circ}$ was added to the flask immersed in a water bath maintained at $37 \pm 0.5^{\circ}$. A three-blade, 5-cm. diameter, polyethylene propeller was inserted through the center opening of the flask and immersed in the dissolution medium to a depth of 27 mm. The propeller was centered and used at a stirring rate of 50 r.p.m. using a constant speed motor.

In each case, microcapsules were placed on the surface of the dissolution medium. At appropriate time intervals, samples of the dissolution medium were withdrawn using a pipet fitted with a cotton plug. A constant volume of the dissolution medium was maintained by the addition of an equal volume of the dissolution medium after each 2 ml. sample was withdrawn. In each case, the cotton plug was added to the dissolution mixture. Concentrations were determined spectrophtometrically after appropriate dilutions were made. All analyses were made spectrophtometrically at 240 nm. using appropriate blanks and standards.

## Results and Discussion

The dissolution rate profiles of microcapsules prepared with unfractionated gelatin and gelatin fractions at pH 3.7 are shown in Fig. 1. In this figure, the dissolution rate profile of unencapsulated phenobarbital particles has also been included for comparison purposes.

In a situation where different molecular weight fractions of a gelatin are used for preparing microcapsules under identical conditions, one would expect that there would be some sort of correlation between the release patterns of the microcapsules and the gelatin molecular weight used for preparing the particular microcapsules. Results found in Fig. 1, however, do not show this type of correlation. The release profiles show that the microcapsules prepared with fraction III had the slowest release rate followed by fractions II < I < IV.

Comparing the release profiles of microcapsules in Fig. 1 with the wall thickness of microcapsules in Table III, it is found that the release rates of microcapsules were dependent on the wall thickness. Microcapsules prepared with gelatin fractions producing thicker walls were found to yield slower release profile.

The type of results obtained as found in Fig. 1 suggests two possibilities: (i) the gelatin fractions are extremely dissimilar having markedly different characteristics, or (ii) the gelatin fractions, though identical in nature, differed in the availability of salt-bond forming linkages or had different optimum pH of coacervation, or both. The former of the two possibilities seems very much remote, since it has been shown by a number of investigators (1, 4, 36) that fractionation by coacervation yields homogeneous fractions. It is therefore more probable that the gelatin fractions were identical in nature, but differed either in the availability of salt-bond forming linkages, or had different optimum pH of coacervation, or both. In either case, changing the pH of preparation of microcapsules would be one way of finding it out.

In order to study the effect of pH of preparation of microcapsules, it was necessary to know the range of pH where coacervation was taking place. Visual observation with a light microscope showed that coacervation took place between the pH

TABLE I
FRACTIONATION OF GELATIN

| Gelatin Fraction | Acetone:Water Ratio | Percent in Fraction | Isoionic Point |
|---|---|---|---|
| Fraction I | 0.90 | 45 | $8.40 \pm 0.2$ |
| Fraction II | 0.95 | 19 | $8.45 \pm 0.2$ |
| Fraction III | 1.05 | 21 | $8.50 \pm 0.2$ |
| Fraction IV | 1.15 | 10 | $8.45 \pm 0.2$ |

TABLE II
INTRINSIC VISCOSITIES [a] OF GELATINS
AND MOLECULAR WEIGHTS [b] OF GELATIN FRACTIONS

| Gelatin Fraction | Intrinsic Viscosity | Minimum Molecular Weight | Weight-Average Molecular Weight |
|---|---|---|---|
| Fraction I | 1.05 | 116,000 | 281,000 |
| Fraction II | 0.85 | 78,000 | 239,000 |
| Fraction III | 0.51 | 62,000 | 137,000 |
| Fraction IV | 0.44 | 59,000 | 118,000 |

(a) Each value is an average of at least three determinations.
(b) Determined by Analytical Ultracentrifuge.
(c) Extrapolated from Fig.

TABLE III
CORRELATION OF WALL THICKNESS AND IN VITRO $t_{50}$

| Gelatin Fraction Used for Preparing Microcapsules | pH of Preparation of Microcapsules | Wall Thickness(a) in Microns | In Vitro $t_{50}$ [a] in Minutes |
|---|---|---|---|
| I | 3.2 | 3.01 | 44 |
| I | 3.7 | 3.84 | 50 |
| I | 4.2 | 2.60 | 41.5 |
| II | 3.7 | 6.01 | 61.5 |
| III | 3.2 | 8.25 | 89 |
| III | 3.7 | 8.56 | 97 |
| III | 4.2 | 6.75 | 71.5 |
| IV | 3.7 | 2.63 | 40 |

(a) Each value is an average of at least three determinations.

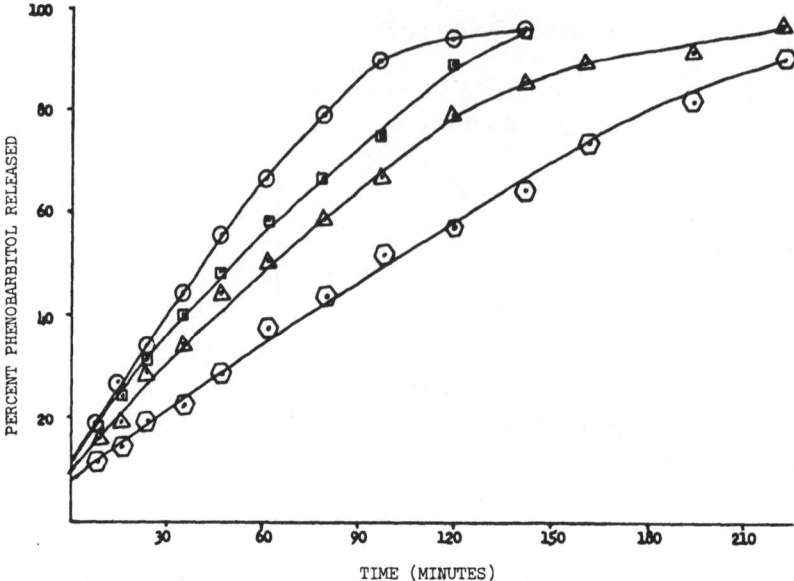

Figure 1.   Release rate of phenobarbital microcapsule pre-
            pared at pH 3.7.
                ⊙Fraction IV      ⊡ Fraction I      ▲ Fraction II
                ◉ Fraction III

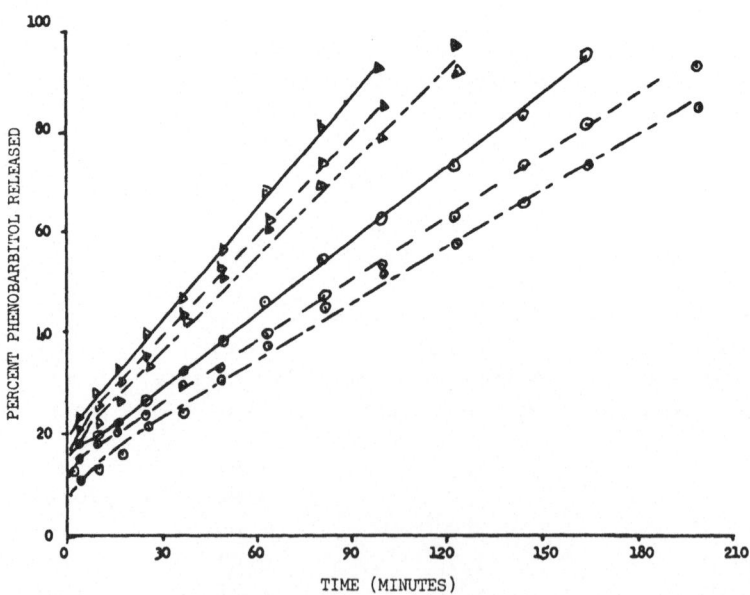

Figure 2.   Release rate of phenobarbital microcapsules as
            a function of pH of preparation
                △ Fraction I        ◯ Fraction III
            ——— pH 4.2    – – – – pH 3.2    –·–·– pH 3.7

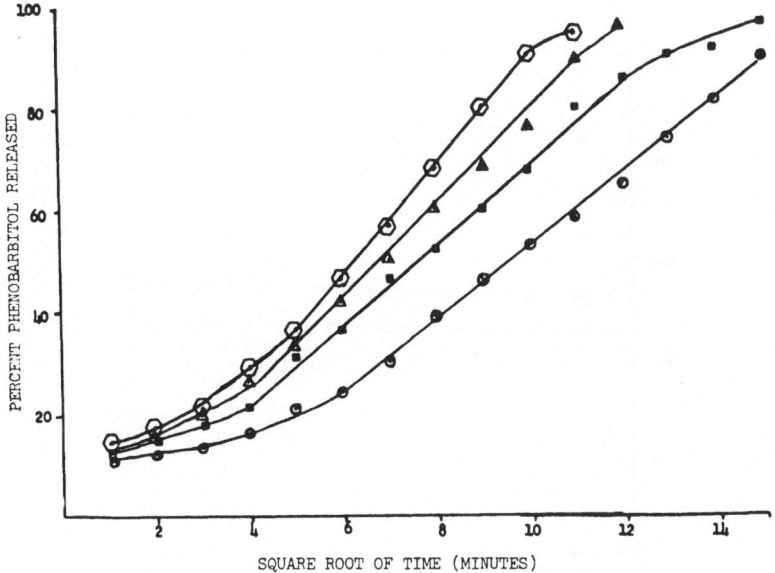

Figure 3.   Percent phenobarbital released as a function
of square root of time (pH of preparation of
microcapsules = 3.7).

　　　　⬡ Fraction IV　　　△ Fraction I

　　　　▢ Fraction II　　　◯ Fraction III

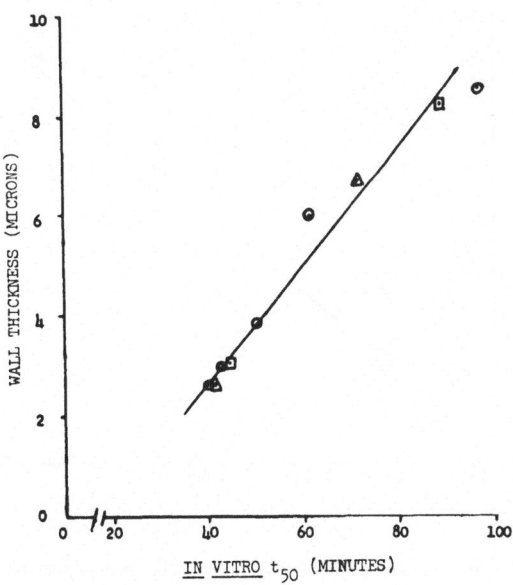

Figure 4.   _In_ _Vitro_ $t_{50}$ as a function of wall thickness.

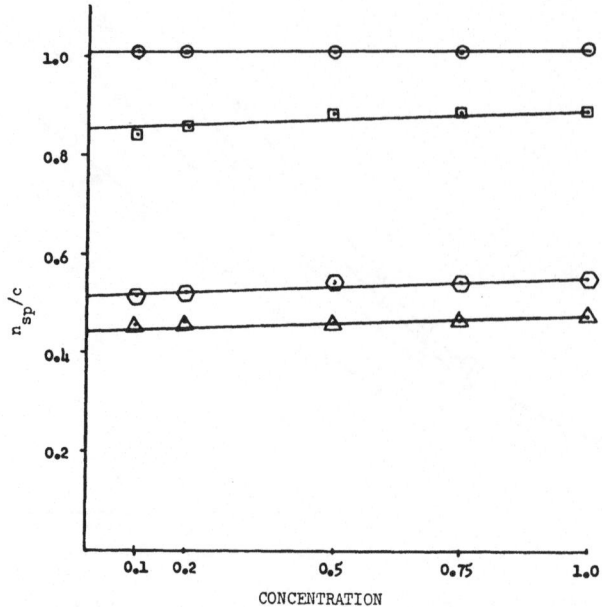

Figure 5.  Intrinsic Viscosity of Gelation Fractions.

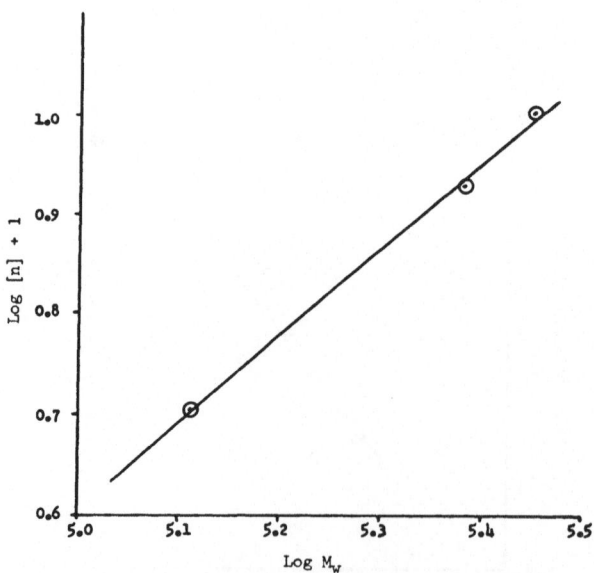

Figure 6.   Log molecular weight as a function of
            log intrinsic viscosity.

values of 2.5 and 4.5.   Therefore, pH values of 3.2 and 4.2
were selected for further examination since these values were
well within the range of coacervation in the system being studied.

The gelatin fractions selected for studying the effect of pH
of preparation were fractions I and III, since, as shown in Fig.
1, microcapsules prepared with these fractions at pH 3.7 exhibited the faster and slower rates respectively.

Fig. 2 shows the release profiles of microcapsules prepared with gelatin fractions I and III at pH 3.2 and at pH 4.2.
The results indicate the same trend of release pattern as was
observed when the capsules were prepared at pH 3.7.   The release rates of microcapsules prepared with gelatin fractions I
and III at pH 3.2 are almost identical to those of microcapsules
prepared at pH 3.7.   On the other hand, the capsules prepared
at pH 4.2 show faster release rates compared to the ones prepared at pH 3.7 in both cases.

Similar release patterns at pH 3.2 and pH 3.7 suggest
that coacervation was maximum in this region of pH, whereas
faster release rates at pH 4.2 indicate a diminishing tendency
toward coacervation as the pH of preparation of microcapsules
is increased.   In the light of these results, it would appear that
the optimum pH of coacervation as well as tendency toward
coacervation for both gelatin fractions I and III was similar or
very nearly so.

The similarity of the trend of release patterns observed
with release profiles of microcapsules prepared at pH 3.2,
3.7, and 4.2 also suggest that the gelatin fractions were neither
dissimilar nor did they have markedly different characteristics.
If the gelatin fractions were dissimilar, then the release rate
patterns would have shown different trends when the pH of
preparation was changed.

Therefore it appears that the gelatin fractions were indeed identical in nature.   This view is further strengthened from
the results of isoionic point determination, since, dissimilar
fractions of gelatin would be more likely to show a markedly
different isoionic point for each fraction.   These results therefore strongly suggest that the gelatin fractions were neither
dissimilar nor did they have a markedly different optimum pH
of coacervation, and that the differences observed in the release

rates were most probably due to the differences in the availability of salt-forming linkages in each fraction.

In their study on the molecular configuration of gelatin, Veis and Cohen (6) examined two commercial gelatins of approximately the same molecular weights. The gelatins used were an acid-precursor pigskin gelatin and an alkali-precursor calf-skin gelatin. Light scattering and viscosity measurements in dilute salt solution and under salt-free isoionic conditions indicated that acid-precursor gelatin did not show marked configurational changes nor the pronounced intermolecular attraction in isoionic solutions as compared to alkali-precursor gelatin.

Veis et al. (7) extended this line of investigation and showed by light scattering and electrophoretic mobility studies as a function of pH that unlike alkali-precursor gelatins, acid-precursor gelatins did not exhibit sharply defined changes in properties in the region of the isoelectric point. Conductivity measurements of Carr and Topol (40) showed that small ions were bound by the acid-precursor gelatin in the pH 6-9 range, while no salt was bound by the alkali-precursor gelatin in the region of isoelectric point (pH 5). Similarly, Bello et al. (41) showed that many salts shifted the pH of solutions of an acid-precursor gelatin. Pouradier (39) also noted the same anomaly, in that the low molecular weight acid-precursor calf-skin gelatin fractions showed a decrease in the number of free carboxyl groups as compared to the number of such groups per unit weight in higher molecular weight gelatin fractions, thereby indicating differences in the number of chains per molecule.

All of these studies (6, 7, 37-41) indicate that the low molecular weight gelatin fractions carry larger number of chains per molecule compared to high molecular weight fractions which not only carry relatively smaller number of chains per molecule but are also compact structures formed in such a way as to provide for the proximity of oppositely charged functional groups. In the light of these studies, then, it is quite reasonable to believe that the low molecular weight fractions of gelatin had relatively larger number of salt-bond forming sites available for interaction with the oppositely charged acacia particles. The dissolution patterns as found in Figures 1 and 2 confirm this hypothesis since the release rates of phenobarbital reduced with decreasing molecular weights of gelatin fractions used for preparing the microcapsules. However, microcapsules

made with fraction IV do not show this trend. One reason for
this indifferent behaviour of microcapsules made with fraction
IV may be that the electrostatic interaction in this particular
case was not strong enough. Either the chain lengths were too
small, or the coacervate droplets had difficulty adhering to the
phenobarbital particles, or both. This view is further strengthened by recalling the work of Saunders and Ward (10, 42).

In a study aimed at elucidating the physical properties of
gelatin and its degradation products, Saunders and Ward (42)
studied the structures of gels of a series of fractions of a high
grade gelatin (pI = 4. 95). Examination of gel structures
measured in terms of rigidity confirmed their previous findings
(10) that, above $M_w$ = 60, 000 the regidity of gels prepared from
fractions slightly decreased with increasing molecular weight
and marked similarities in the structure of gels, by the approxi-
mate constancy of the gel rigidity, were observed. The authors
(42) extended their study to examine the strain dependence of
the modulus of rigidity by the concentric cylinder apparatus.
The rigidity modulus was determined at small (low) strain in
the range 0. 12 to 0. 2 and also at large strain in the range 0. 2
to 0. 8. In both cases the usual rigidity plateau was found to be
falling away when $M_w$ was less than 60, 000. The authors (42)
concluded from these results that there was a critical molecular
weight of 60, 000 and only above this value there was substantial
independence of gel properties with respect to molecular weight.

An attempt to explain the mechanism of release of medicaments incorporated into solid matrices has been made by a
number of investigators (43-47). It has been shown that the release of medicaments from such systems may be considered as
taking place through simple diffusional process or through
leaching by dissolution into the permeating fluid, or both.

Higuchi (43, 44) developed theoretical equations to explain
the release of medicaments from homogeneous matrix by simple
diffusional process and from a granular matrix for the leaching
type release mechanism occuring through diffusion movement
utilizing intergranular openings.

When a spherical pellet is used, the release of medicament by diffusional process into a bathing medium acting essentially as a perfect sink is given by the equation:

$$1 - 3\left(\frac{a_1}{a_o}\right)^2 + 2\left(\frac{a_1}{a_o}\right)^3 = \frac{6 \, D \, C_s}{A \, a_o^2} \, t$$

where D = the diffusivity of the drug in the permeating fluid

$C_s$ = the solubility of the drug in the permeating fluid

A = the total amount of drug in the permeating fluid

$a_o$ = the radius of the whole pellet

$a_1$ = the radius of that part still unextracted at time t.

Where A    $C_s$, the fraction of drug remaining in the pellet = $(a_1/a_o)^3$.

Similarly, for a spherical pellet the equation for release of medicament through leaching by the external solvent is given as:

$$1 - 3\left(\frac{a_1}{a_o}\right)^2 + 2\left(\frac{a_1}{a_o}\right)^3 = \frac{6 \, D \, C_s}{A \, a_o^2} \frac{E - E_o}{T} \, t$$

where T = the tortuosity factor of the capillar system

E = porosity of the leached portion of the pellet

$E_o$ = initial porosity of the initially formed matrix

and the remaining symbols have the same meaning as described above. Again, the residual fraction = $(a_1/a_o)^3$. In this case the drug is presumed to dissolve slowly into the permeating fluid phase and to diffuse from the system along the cracks and capillary channels filled with the extracting solvent. In this instance, the intragranular diffusion is assumed to be insignificant.

From these two equations it can be seen that in either case a plot of residual fraction $(a_1/a_o)^3$ as a function of square root of time should yield a straight line. A number of investigations (48-51) have shown linear square root of time plots.

Fig. 3 is a plot of percent phenobarbital released as a function of square root of time for microcapsules prepared at pH 3.7. The plot is linear over a wide range (between 25% and 85% phenobarbital released) for capsules made with unfractionated gelatin and all gelatin fractions studied. The terminal ends of the plot, i.e., those portions of the plot which represent the

first 25% and the last 15% of phenobarbital released are not
linear however, but do show the release rate patterns of Figs. 1
and 2 in a somewhat better form.

The portion of the graph representing the initial 25% phenobarbital released shows what appears to be a large initial surge of
release followed by a slower rate of release. The large initial
surge of release accounts for the first 10 to 15 percent phenobarbital released almost as soon as the dissolution determinations were started. This could be due to some phenobarbital
retained within the wall material during the process of encapsulation and/or phenobarbital entrapped in or on the wall material
during treatment with isopropanol due to solvent migration
effect, and which dissolved rather quickly in the dissolution
medium almost as soon as the microcapsules came in contact
with the dissolution medium. This is followed by a slow rate
of release up to the point represented by about 25% phenobarbital released. This could be due to what may be called a short
lag time required to wet the capsules or the interior of the
matrix, or both. Once the period of initial surge and the lag
time required to wet the capsules is over, the dissolution follows
a linear relationship up to the point when 85% to 90% of phenobarbital has been released.

The last portion of Fig. 3 representing the final 10-15
percent phenobarbital released shows that the release rate
started to decrease appreciably. This could be due to a number
of reasons: (i) at this point there is not enough phenobarbital
left to dissolve, (ii) after the initial dissolution of most of
phenobarbital, a sort of hollow portion is created between the
matrix and the very small portion of the undissolved phenobarbital particle and the surface area of this small residual portion
of the undissolved phenobarbital is not sufficient to maintain a
high concentration of phenobarbital solution inside the shell to
maintain the required concentration gradient. Either one or a
combination of these factors would have a tendency to slow down
the release rate appreciably.

Among the various factors on which the success of microencapsulation procedure depends, wall thickness of the encapsulating material is perhaps one of the most important (1).
Wagner (52) has suggested that the time for 50% of the drug to
dissolve in vitro ($t50\%$) is probably the best in vitro variable to
correlate since: (i) its value indicates the central tendency of

the in vitro dissolution data and (ii) by use of this value one has
not commited oneself to any formal kinetic interpretation of the
data.   The $t_{50\%}$ of the various microcapsules were therefore
determined from Figs. 1 and 2 in order to correlate the wall
thickness of the encapsulating material.   The data has been
tabulated in Table III and plotted in Fig. 4 and it is clear from
the results found in Table III and Fig. 4 that the wall thickness
of the microcapsules was directly related to the in vitro $t_{50\%}$
in all cases examined.

## REFERENCES

1.   A. Veis, E. Bodor, and S. Mussel, Biopolymers, 5,
     37(1967).
2.   A. Veis, J. Cohen, J. Am. Chem. Soc. 78, 6238(1956).
3.   A. Veis, J. Anesey, and J. Cohen, J. Am. Leather
     Chemists' Assoc., 55, 548(1960).
4.   A. Veis, J. Phys. Chem., 67, 1960(1963).
5.   G. Scatchard, J. L. Oncley, J. W. Williams, and A.
     Brown, J. Am. Chem. Soc., 66, 1980(1944).
6.   A. Veis and J. Cohen, J. Polymer Sci., 26, 113 (1957).
7.   A. Veis, J. Anesey, and J. Cohen, in "Recent Advances
     in Gelatin and Glue Research", G. Stainsby, Ed., Perga-
     mon Press, New York, 1958, p. 155.
8.   J. Pouradier and A. M. Venet, J. Chim. Phys., 47,
     11(1950).
9.   G. Stainsby, Discussions Faraday Soc., 18, 288(1954).
10.  G. Stainsby, P. R. Saunders, and A. G. Ward, J.
     Polymer Sci., 12, 325(1954).
11.  P. L. Madan, M. S. Thesis, University of Georgia, Athens,
     Georgia 1971.
12.  P. L. Madan, L. A. Luzzi, and J. C. Price, J. Pharm.
     Sci., 61 1586(1972).
13.  L. A. Luzzi and R. J. Gerraughty, J. Pharm. Sci., 53,
     429(1964).
14.  L. A. Luzzi and R. J. Gerraughty, J. Pharm. Sci., 56,
     634(1967).
15.  L. A. Luzzi and R. J. Gerraughty, J. Pharm. Sci., 56
     1174(1967).
16.  B. K. Green and L. Schleiker, U. S. patent,
     2,730,456 (1956).
17.  B. K. Green and L. Schleiker, U. S. patent,
     2,730,457 (1956).
18.  B. K. Green and L. Schleiker, U. S. patent,
     2,800,457 (1957).

19.  Erick H. Jensen and John G. Wagner, U. S. patent
     3, 069, 370 (1962).
20.  B. K. Green, U. S. patent 2, 712, 507 (1955).
21.  Jerrold L. Anderson, Gary L. Gardner and Noble H.
     Yoshida, U. S. patent 3, 341, 416 (1967).
22.  Robert Erwin Miller and Jerrold L. Anderson, U. S.
     patent 3, 155, 590 (1964).
23.  J. C. Hecker and O. D. Hawks, U. S. patent 3, 137, 630
     (1964).
24.  Gerhard Levy, Jack R. Leonards and Josephine A.
     Procknal, J. Pharm. Sci. , 54, 1719 (1965).
25.  H. C. Caldwell and E. Rosen, J. Pharm. Sci. , 53,
     1387 (1964).
26.  C. Brynko, J. A. Bakan, R. E. Miller and J. A. Scarpelli,
     U. S. patent, 3, 341, 466 (1967).
27.  J. R. Nixon, Saleh, A. H. Khalil, and J. E. Carless, J.
     Pharm. Pharmc. , 20, 528 (1968).
28.  S. N. Luu, P. F. Carlier, P. Delort, J. Gazzola, and
     D. LaFont, J. Pharm. Sci. , 62, 452 (1973).
29.  E. O. Kraemer, J. Phys. Chem. , 45, 660 (1941).
30.  H. Boedtker and P. Doty, J. Phys. Chem. , 58, 968 (1954).
31.  H. Boedtker and P. Doty, J. Am. Chem. Soc. , 78, 4267
     (1956).
32.  D. C. Carpenter and J. J. Kucera, J. Phys. Chem. , 35,
     2619 (1931).
33.  D. C. Carpenter, A. C. Dahlberg, and J. C. Henning,
     Ind. Eng. Chem.
34.  D. C. Carpenter, Cold Spring Harbor Symposia Quant.
     Biol. , 6, 244 (1938).
35.  T. W. Underwood and D. E. Cadwallader, J. Pharm. Sci. ,
     61, 239 (1972).
36.  J. Pouradier and A. M. Venet, J. Chim. Phys. , 47, 391
     (1950).
37.  A. Courts, Biochem. J. , 58, 70 (1954).
38.  A. Courts and G. Stainsby, in "R ecent Advances in Gelatin
     and Glue Research", G. Stainsby, Ed. , Pergamon Press,
     New York, 1958, p. 100.
39.  J. Pouradier, in "Recent Advances in Gelatin and Glue
     Research", G. Stainsby, Ed. , Pergamon Press, New
     York, 1958, p. 265.
40.  C. W. Carr and L. Topol, J. Phys. Chem. , 54, 176(1950).
41.  J. Bello, H. C. A. Riese, and J. R. Vinograd, J. Phys.
     Chem. , 60, 1299 (1956).

42.    P. R. Saunders and A. G. Ward, in "Recent Advances in Gelatin Glue Research", G. Stainsby, Ed., Pergamon Press, New York 1958, p. 197.
43.    T. Higuchi, J. Pharm. Sci., 50, 874 (1961).
44.    T. Higuchi, J. Pharm. Sci., 52, 1145 (1963).
45.    J. G. Wagner, Drug. Std., 27, 178 (1959).
46.    R. G. Wiegand and J. D. Taylor, Drug. Std., 27, 165 (1959).
47.    H. W. Mattson, Intern. Science Technol., p. 66 (1956).
48.    S. J. Desai, A. P. Simonelli, and W. I. Higuchi, J. Pharm. Sci., 54, 1459 (1956).
49.    S. J. Desai, P. Singh, A. P. Simonelli, and W. Higuchi, J. Pharm., Sci., 55, 1335 (1966).
50.    S. J. Desai, P. Singh, A. P. Simonelli, and W. Higuchi, J. Pharm. Sci., 55, 1230 (1966).
51.    S. J. Desai, P. Singh, A. P. Simonelli and W. Higuchi, J. Pharm. Sci., 55, 1235 (1966).
52.    J. G. Wagner, in "Biopharmaceutics and Relevent Pharmacokinetics", Drug Intelligence Publications, Hamilton, Ill., 1971, p. 213.

# ENCAPSULATED VEGETABLE FATS IN CATTLE FEEDS

Joel Bitman, T. R. Wrenn, L. P. Dryden, L. F. Edmondson
and R. A. Yoncoskie
Biochemistry Laboratory, Beltsville, Maryland   20705
and Dairy Products Laboratory, Washington, D. C.   20250
Agricultural Research Service
U. S. Department of Agriculture

Atherosclerosis is the major specific type of heart disease afflicting mankind.  It is characterized by an accumulation of fatty materials, particularly cholesterol, in the walls of medium and large arteries.  Human populations consuming diets high in saturated fats and cholesterol have high serum cholesterol levels and high mortality rates from heart disease (1).  Cardiovascular disease is the cause of about  50 per cent of deaths in men 40 to 60 years old in the United States.  Studies of risk factors for coronary heart disease in the American male population have documented increased incidence rates with increasing serum cholesterol levels (1). Epidemiologic studies in seven countries demonstrated that populations consuming diets high in saturated fats had high mortality rates from coronary heart disease (2).  Death rates for middle-aged American men were over four times greater than for countries whose population had low percentages of their dietary calories coming from saturated fats.

About 3 years ago the Inter-Society Commission for Heart Disease Resources recommended that the nation's food producing industry make a major effort to change the type of fat people eat (1).  They recommended a reduction in saturated fat of animal products and an increased consumption of polyunsaturated fats.  Thus, there will be increasing public pressures to do at least three things: (a) reduce the overall consumption of fats, (b) lower the amount of fat in foods, and (c) change the nature of the fat in food.

The United States Department of Agriculture is concerned about this problem and our research has been directed toward finding ways in which the polyunsaturated fat content of milk and meat can be

JOEL BITMAN ET AL.

increased. The plant fat which ruminants ingest is primarily
polyunsaturated, but meat and milk fat normally contain only 2-4%
polyunsaturated fat. The data in Table 1 show that the major fatty
acid in grass is linolenic acid but in the rumen, microorganisms
hydrogenate the polyunsaturated fatty acids of the plant fat.

About three years ago Australian scientists developed a technique
to increase polyunsaturated fats (4). They enclosed polyunsaturated
vegetable oils in a protein coat and then treated the protein coat
with formaldehyde, thus protecting the polyunsaturated fat from the
bacteria in the rumen. The formaldehyde-protein coat is stable in
the neutral conditions (pH 6-7) of the rumen. After hydrolysis in
the lower digestive tract under the more acidic conditions existing
in the abomasum and the intestine, the polyunsaturated fat is
digested and absorbed, thereby resulting in higher amounts of
polyunsaturated fats in milk (4) and in meat (5).

We have used this encapsulated oil technique during the last
two years to produce polyunsaturated milk, cheese, veal and beef (6,7).
This paper reviews our research on the "protected" feed technique of
modifying milk and meat fats.

TABLE 1

Fatty Acid Composition of Pasture Grass and
Bovine Milk and Meat Fat[a]

| Fatty acid | | Weight % in lipid | | |
|---|---|---|---|---|
| | | Grass | Milk | Meat |
| Myristic | 14:0 | 1 | 12 | 3 |
| Palmitic | 16:0 | 11 | 31 | 26 |
| Stearic | 18:0 | 2 | 11 | 14 |
| Oleic | 18:1 | 5 | 24 | 47 |
| Linoleic | 18:2 | 12 | 3 | 3 |
| Linolenic | 18:3 | 62 | 1 | 1 |
| Others | | 7[b] | 18[c] | 6[d] |

[a]Source of data: grass (3); milk and meat fat-present study.

[b]Primarily 12:0 and 16:1.

[c]4:0-12:0 Comprise 11%; 14:1 and 16:1, 4%; minor acids, 3%.

[d]Primarily 16:1.

## MATERIALS AND METHODS

### Preparation of Feed Supplements

Encapsulation, or "protection", is accomplished by coating finely dispersed oil droplets with a formaldehyde-treated protein, or other crosslinked polymer combinations.  The crosslinked coating resists breakdown in the rumen of animals.  Several techniques of blending mixtures of vegetable oils, protein solutions and formalin, or treating oil seed fractions with formalin, and processing into a suitable feed supplement have been studied.  Most of the work done to date, both in Australia and in ARS laboratories, has been carried out by feeding a spray dried formalin-treated emulsion of soidum caseinate and vegetable oil.

### Spray-Dried Oil-Caseinate Emulsion

Spray dried protected supplement was prepared by homogenizing a vegetable oil with a solution of sodium caseinate (about 10 percent casein heated to 70°C), treating with formalin (6 to 8 percent by weight of protein) and spray drying.  We have formulated most of the lots of this supplement with an oil:casein ration of 2:1.  Both formalin and the vegetable oil may be metered into a continuous flow line of the caseinate solution before homogenizing; alternatively, for small lots, the oil may be added to the caseinate solution in a vat and then homogenized.  In the latter case, formalin was added slowly to the homogenized blend with thorough stirring.

### Protected Supplement from Soybeans

Ground whole soybeans (<3mm) were mixed in a horizontal feed mixer for 66 hr with a 37% formaldehyde solution (ca 10% of soybean weight).  The soybean-formaldehyde mixture was dried in a forced air oven at 60°C and attained constant weight after 20 hr.  Full-fat soy flour mixed with 15% of its weight of 37% formaldehyde solution was tumbled and agitated for 18 hr in a liquid-solid blender.  Full-fat soy flakes were treated in a similar manner.  Full-fat soy flour was also homogenized with a whey solution, treated with formaldehyde and spray dried.

### Glutaraldehyde-Treated Gelatin:Gum Arabic Protected Oil

We have prepared a feed supplement in our laboratory by mixing safflower oil with an aqueous solution (50°C) of gum arabic and gelatin, followed by homogenization, adjustment of pH to 4.5 with

sodium hydroxide, cooling, and finally addition of glutaraldehyde
as the crosslinking agent.  This formulation was held overnight
with continuous stirring and spray dried.  This procedure has some
advantages over the oil:caseinate procedure described above.  Its
bulk density was much greater than the caseinate coated material,
which allowed easier mixing with basic feed rations.  It can be
prepared with a higher oil content (85 percent compared to about 65
percent for the caseinate coated material).  Although gelatin was
about as expensive as caseinate, it comprised only about 7.5
percent of the total formula compared to about 33 percent caseinate
in the first described procedure.

## Analytical Procedures

Lipid extracts of milk were prepared by extraction with chloro-
form-methanol (2:1).  Fatty acid esters prepared by the method of
Christopherson and Glass (8) were determined by programmed gas
liquid chromatography on 15% EGS (ethylene glycol succinate) on
Anakrom AB (110/110 mesh) or 10% EGSS-X on gas chrom P (100/120 mesh)
in glass columns with a Model 7621 Hewlett-Packard automated gas
chromatograph.  Milk samples were analyzed for percent fat and
cholesterol (9).  Blood samples were analyzed for cholesterol (9),
triglycerides (10) and nonesterified fatty acids (11).  Adipose
tissue from the tailhead were also analyzed for fatty acids.
Formaldehyde was determined (12) by a modification of the method of
Swain et al. (13) involving hydrolysis with phosphoric acid and
distillation.

## ANIMALS AND TREATMENTS

Mature lactating Holstein cows were fed 200-3200 g per day of
the various supplements as a partial replacement for grain on a w/w
basis.  Four 4-day old Holstein bull calves were fed 6.35 kg/day of
polyunsaturated milk and four control calves were fed the same
quantity of normal milk until 10 weeks of age (14).  Grain and hay
were fed ad libitum.  From 11-18 weeks the calves were fed a ration
which included either formaldehyde protected safflower oil-casein
(SOC-F) or unprotected safflower oil-casein (SOC).  The calves were
slaughtered at 18 weeks of age.  The polyunsaturated and normal beef
were obtained from the Ruminant Nutrition Laboratory, Beltsville,
Maryland (15).  Steers had been fed a ration containing either 10%
or 20% SOC-F or SOC for six weeks.  Cheddar cheese was prepared from
the polyunsaturated milk by the time schedule method (16).

## RESULTS AND DISCUSSION

An increase in the linoleic acid content of milk fat resulted from the inclusion of safflower oil-casein-formaldehyde in the diet of cows (Table 2).  A rapid increase was observed in linoleic acid, from 3% of the total fatty acids at the beginning of an experiment or during control diet feeding, to as much as 30-35% at the top intake level.  The increase was found to be dose dependent (Exp. 2, Table 2).  The major acids showing a compensatory decline were palmitic, 16:0, which decreased from 35% to 14% and myristic, 14:0, which declined from 13% to 4% as the SOC-F level increased from 0 to 2278 g per day.  The simultaneous increase in polyunsaturated fatty acids and lowering of the saturated fatty acids of milk fat are two desirable features recommended for dietary control of heart disease.

TABLE 2

Percent Linoleic Acid in Milk Fat of Cows Fed
Protected or Unprotected Safflower Oil

| Exp | Dietary Material | Days | Amount Fed, g/ day | Percent C18:2 in Milk |
|-----|------------------|------|--------------------|-----------------------|
| 1   | SOC-F            | 5    | 1500               | 33                    |
|     | SOC              | 5    | 1500               | 3                     |
| 2   | SOC-F            | 7    | 0                  | 3                     |
|     | SOC-F            | 7    | 200                | 7                     |
|     | SOC-F            | 7    | 400                | 10                    |
|     | SOC-F            | 7    | 762                | 17                    |
|     | SOC-F            | 7    | 1600               | 24                    |
|     | SOC-F            | 7    | 2278               | 33                    |
| 3   | SOC-F            | 112  | 0                  | 3                     |
|     | SOC-F            | 112  | 800                | 13                    |

SOC-F = Safflower oil-casein formaldehyde.
SOC   = Safflower oil-casein.

The results of the experiments using soybean preparations in attempts to produce polyunsaturated milk more economically are shown in Table 3.  The 18:2 content of the milk increased in each experiment, although the increases were modest.  The encapsulated formaldehyde-treated whey protein-full-fat soy flour was most successful in producing polyunsaturated milk.

TABLE 3

Percent Linoleic Acid in Milk Fat of Cows Fed
Protected or Unprotected Soybean Preparations

| Exp | Dietary Material | Days | Amount Fed, g/day | Percent C18:2 in Milk |
|-----|------------------|------|-------------------|------------------------|
| 1 | SB-F | 3 | 3200 | 6.1 |
| 2 | FFS Flour-F | 6 | 1900 | 3.5 |
|   | FFS Flour | 6 | 1900 | 2.5 |
| 3 | FFS Flakes-F | 3 | 2000 | 4.5 |
|   | FFS Flakes | 3 | 2000 | 2.5 |
| 4 | FFS Flour-W-F | 5 | 3100 | 8.0 |

SB-F=Soybeans-Formaldehyde.
FFS-Flour-F = Full-fat Soy Flour Formaldehyde.
FFS Flour = Full Fat Soy Flour.
FFS Flakes-F = Full Fat Soy Flakes Formaldehyde.
FFS Flakes = Full Fat Soy Flakes.
FFS Flour-W-F = Full Fat Soy Flour-Whey Formaldehyde.

   The relative failure of the soybean-formaldehyde preparations
suggests the possibility that the natural protein does not
encapsulate the oil in the soybeans in the way that casein does in
the safflower oil-casein homogenization procedure.  Electron
photomicrographs were used to evaluate differences between
these preparations.

   The encapsulated vegetable oil produced by the coacervate
process using two proteins, gum arabic and gelatin, was fed to two
cows in two different experiments (Table 4).  Six-fold increases in
C18:2 in the milk fat were observed.  Fig. 1 and Fig. 2 demonstrate
that milk from cows fed the coacervate protected feed exhibited a
rapid increase in linoleic acid to 10-16% of the total fatty acids.
The decline to the control period 3 to 4% linoleic acid was slow
and was not achieved until three days after removal of the protected
fat.  This pattern of rapid rise and carryover was very similar to
that previously seen with the spray-dried oil-caseinate emulsion (6,7).

TABLE 4

Percent Linoleic Acid in Milk Fat of Cows Fed Glutaraldehyde-
Treated Gelatin:Gum Arabic Protected Safflower Oil

| Exp | Days | Amount Fed, g/day | Percent C18:2 in Milk |
|-----|------|-------------------|-----------------------|
| 1   | 5    | 0                 | 2.5                   |
|     | 5    | 800               | 14.3                  |
| 2   | 5    | 0                 | 1.9                   |
|     | 5    | 1000              | 11.2                  |

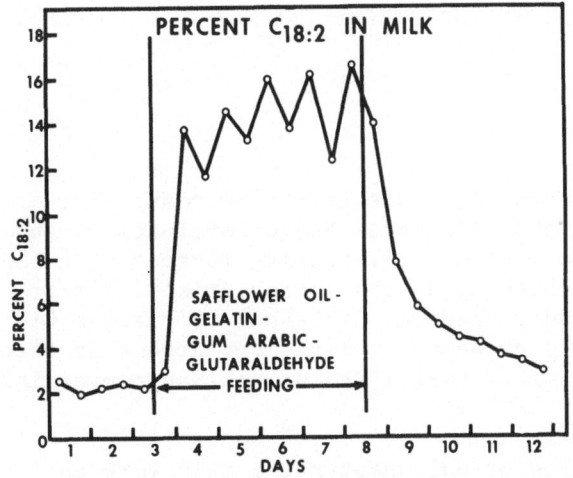

Fig. 1.  Effect of feeding glutaraldehyde-treated
gelatin:gum arabic protected safflower oil on
content of linoleic acid in milk fat.

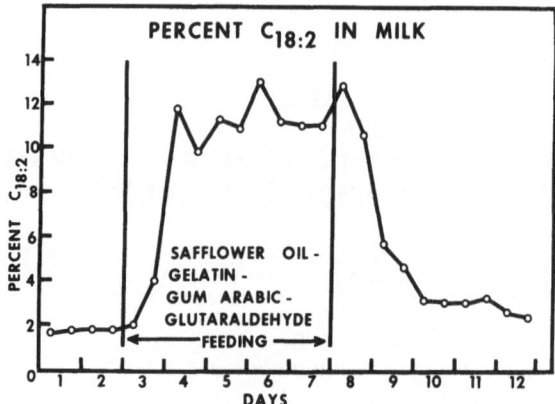

Fig. 2.  Effect of feeding glutaraldehyde-treated gelatin:gum
arabic protected safflower oil on content of linoleic
acid in milk fat.

Cheddar cheeses were made from milk containing 2.4 to 31.7
percent C18:2 in the milk fat.  Flavor evaluations showed a decrease
in the flavor score with corresponding increases in the level of C18:2
(16).  As the cheeses aged, the characteristic flavors became less
noticeable.  Cheddar cheeses with about 15 percent C18:2 in the fat
were of acceptable consumer quality, and processed cheeses with up
to 10-12 percent C18:2 were liked as well as commercially processed
cheese.

Pooled samples of polyunsaturated milk were evaluated for
flavor (17).  Flavor scores decreased with increasing amounts of
C18:2.  The off-flavors were predominantly of an oxidized type.  The
oxidized flavor was found to be negligible in raw milk immediately
after milking but increased markedly after 24 hours of refrigerated
storage.  When an anti-oxidant (alpha tocopherol) was added to
freshly drawn milk, the development of off-flavors was prevented.

## Changes in Blood Lipids

Blood cholesterol, triglycerides and nonesterified fatty acids all increased markedly as the cows were fed increasing amounts of SOC-F. The three-fold increase in triglyceride and nonesterified fatty acid probably represents the greater transfer of dietary lipid into the blood. The two-fold increase in cholesterol was interpreted to be an obligatory response to aid in transport of greater amounts of circulating 18:2 fatty acids and total lipids. When the cows were fed SOC-F for 4 months, blood cholesterol was two to three times control levels (Fig. 3). In spite of the very large increase in blood cholesterol in SOC-F fed cows, there was no increase in cholesterol in the milk, indicating a blood-milk barrier for cholesterol (Fig. 4).

## Health Aspects

There were no toxic effects in the ruminants ingesting the dietary supplements containing formaldehyde. Cows have been fed these materials for 8 months with no apparent effects on health, body weight or milk production. Amounts of formaldehyde that we determined in polyunsaturated milk, cheese and meat from animals ingesting formaldehyde-containing feed were similar to amounts found in normal milk, cheese and meat (Table 5). There is no evidence that formaldehyde is transferred into or accumulates in milk and muscle tissue. Our results suggest that much of the small quantity of formaldehyde found in these foods was generated by the acid hydrolytic analytical method.

## Changes in Body Fat Composition

Feeding polyunsaturated milk and SOC-F to calves caused a 4-fold increase in the C18:2 content of the depot fat and cuts of meat (Table 6). The increases observed in linoleic acid concentration of body fat deposits were balanced by compensatory decreases in saturated fatty acids, primarily palmitic (C16:0) and, to a lesser extent, myristic (C14:0). When steers were fed the protected oil ration, carcass fat contained increased amounts of linoleic acid (Table 6). Taste panels rated the polyunsaturated veal and beef in these experiments as equal in flavor, tenderness and juiciness to normal veal and beef.

## Cost Considerations

Reducing the cost of protected feeds is an important aspect of this research and crucial to its success. It has been difficult to evaluate the cost of production of an encapsulated oil-casein-formaldehyde particle as a dietary supplement for milk production

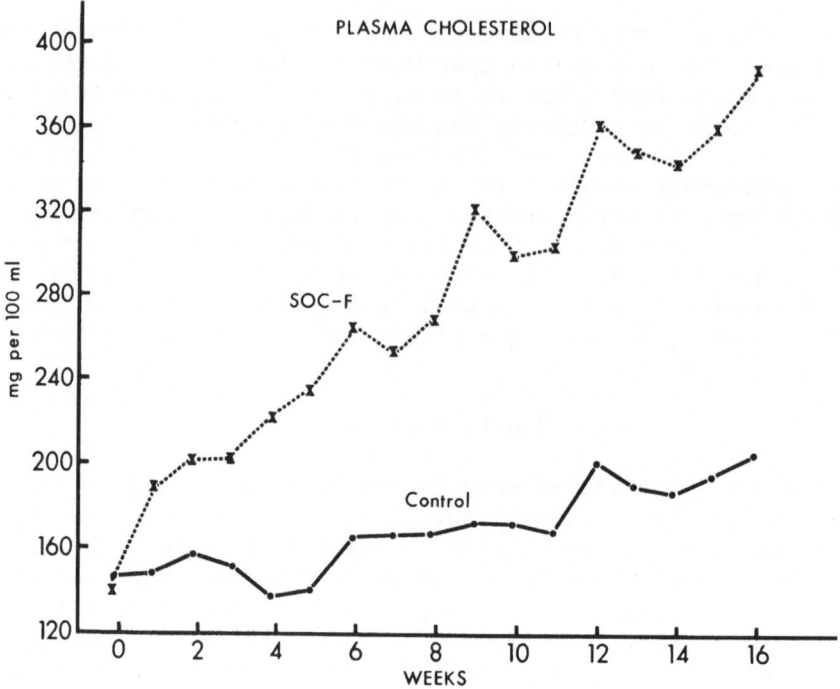

**Fig. 3.  Blood cholesterol during long term SOC-F Feeding.**

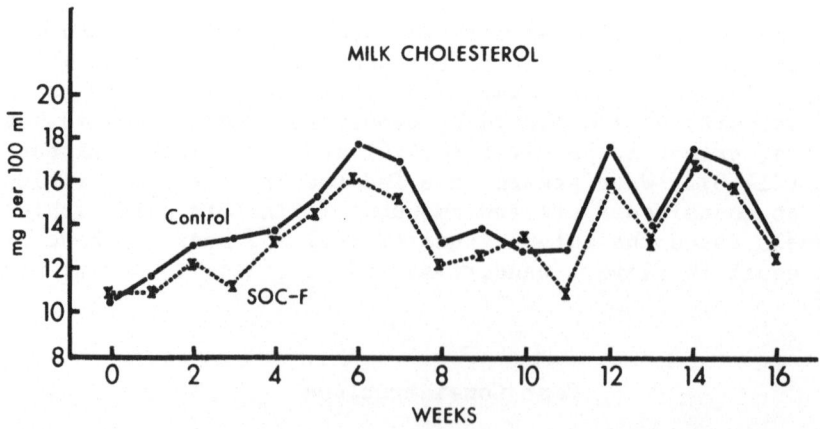

**Fig. 4.  Milk cholesterol during long term SOC-F feeding.**

TABLE 5

Formaldehyde Content of Milk, Cheese and Meat

| Sample | N | ppm | Percent |
|---|---|---|---|
| Milk Herd | 14 | 1.8 | 0.0002 |
| Milk SOC | 15 | 1.9 | 0.0002 |
| Milk SOC-F | 16 | 1.7 | 0.0002 |
| Cheese SOC | 4 | 10 | 0.001 |
| Cheese SOC-F | 5 | 10 | 0.001 |
| Beef SOC | 10 | 39 | 0.004 |
| Beef SOC-F | 5 | 36 | 0.004 |
| Veal SOC | 5 | 100 | 0.010 |
| Veal SOC-F | 4 | 56 | 0.006 |

TABLE 6

Linoleic Acid Content of Depot Fat at Slaughter

| Group | Diet | | Percent C18:2 |
|---|---|---|---|
| Calves | 0-10 wk | 10-18 wk | |
| | NM | SOC | 3.0 |
| | PUM | SOC | 10.2 |
| | NM | SOC-F | 10.9 |
| | PUM | SOC-F | 12.4 |
| Steers | 6 weeks | | |
| | 10% SOC | | 2 |
| | 20% SOC | | 2 |
| | 10% SOC-F | | 13 |
| | 20% SOC-F | | 18 |

NM = Normal Milk.
PUM = Polyunsaturated Milk.

because of several factors.  All feeds used to date have been produced
by highly trained and highly paid scientists usually employing
laboratory or small pilot plant equipment, rather than the larger
industrial type spray dryer.  Costs of the polyunsaturated oils and
casein are also high.  Additionally, any realistic evaluation must
be based upon the value of the resultant polyunsaturated consumer
products, factors which are unknown at this time.

There is not a great likelihood that the preparation of an
encapsulated supplement for feeding to dairy cows to produce polyunsaturated milk can compete economically with direct homogenization
of polyunsaturated oils into skim milk.  While at the present
time there may be certain legal problems to direct addition of
polyunsaturated fats to milk in the processing plant, public
pressures may bring about changes in such restrictions.

Direct synthetic preparation of polyunsaturated cheese and
meat is not presently feasible, however, and the encapsulation
process offers promise therefore, for preparation of these foods.
While the untimate commercial future of these products cannot be
assessed, this method provides a possible means whereby traditional
foods can be produced, consumed and enjoyed by the public without
jeopardy to their health.

## SUMMARY

The technique of increasing the polyunsaturation in milk and
meat fat is still in the experimental stages.  Before its feasibility
can be established, its economic aspects must be studied, more
consistent results must be achieved and an appropriate means must
be found to overcome the tendency of highly unsaturated fats to undergo
oxidative changes.  This research technique involving encapsulation
provides a possible means whereby traditional foods with higher
polyunsaturated fat content can be provided to the public which has
become increasingly concerned with health, heart disease and saturated
fats.

## REFERENCES

1.  "Report of Inter-Society Commission for Heart Disease Resources"
      Circulation 42, December 1970.

2.  Keys, A. ed.  Coronary Heart Disease in Seven Countries.  Ameri-
      can Heart Association.  New York, N. Y , 1970.

3.  Hilditch, T. P. and P. N. Williams, "The Chemical Constitution
      of Natural Fat ", Fourth Edition, John Wiley and Sons, Inc.,
      New York, 1964.

4. Scott, T. W., L. J. Cook, K. A. Ferguson, I. W. McDonald, R. A. Buchanan and G. Loftus Hills. Aust. J. Sci. 32:291, 1970.

5. Faichney, G. F., H. Lloyd Davis, T. W. Scott and L. J. Cook. Aust. J. Biol. Sci. 24:205, 1972.

6. Plowman, R. D., J. Bitman, C. H. Gordon, L. P. Dryden, H. K. Goering, L. F. Edmondson, R. A. Yoncoskie and F. W. Douglas, Jr. J. Dairy Sci. 55:204, 1972.

7. Bitman, J., L. P. Dryden, H. K. Goering, T. R. Wrenn, R. A. Yoncoskie and L. F. Edmondson. J. Am. Oil Chem. Soc. 50:93, 1973.

8. Christopherson, S. W. and R. L. Glass. J. Dairy Sci. 52:1289, 1969.

9. Sobel, A. E. and A. M. Mayer. J. Biol. Chem. 157:255, 1945.

10. Van Handel, E. and D. B. Zilversmit. J. Lab. Clin. Med. 50:152, 1957.

11. Annison, E. F. Aust. J. Agr. Res. 11:58, 1960.

12. Bitman, J., T. R. Wrenn, H. K. Goering, L. P. Dryden and L. F. Edmondson. J. Am. Oil Chem. Soc. 50:93A, 1973.

13. Swain, A. P., E. L. Kokes, N. J. Hipp, J. L. Wood and R. W. Jackson. Ind. Eng. Chem. 40:465, 1948.

14. Wrenn, T. R., J. R. Weyant, C. H. Gordon, H. K. Goering, L. P. Dryden, J. Bitman, R. L. King and M. J. Pallansch. J. Dairy Sci. 55:716, 1972.

15. Agricultural Research 21:14, 1973.

16. Wong, N. P., H. E. Walter, J. H. Vestal, D. E. LaCroix and J. A. Alford. J. Dairy Sci. 55:1331, 1972.

17. Edmondson, L. F., F. W. Douglas, Jr., N. H. Rainey and H. K. Goering. J. Dairy Sci. 55:677, 1972.

# LIQUID/LIQUID EXTRACTIONS CARRIED OUT WITH

# MICROCAPSULE-PACKED COLUMNS

M. Wingard, D. Werkmeister & C. Thies

Materials Research Department

Dayton, Ohio 45409

## Introduction

The concept of microencapsulation has become well known and a variety of processes for preparing microcapsules have been developed(1). Among the wide range of potential capsule applications(2)is the use of microcapsules in various membrane separation processes. Chang(3)and others(4,5)recognized this some time ago and have demonstrated that microcapsules perform effectively in several such processes. The high surface area characteristic of microcapsules and the fact that this surface area is fixed by a thin polymer membrane provide unique separation capabilities. Liquid/liquid extraction processes represent an unexplored class of separation techniques that might also benefit from using microcapsules. The ability of liquid membranes to effect liquid/liquid separations has been demonstrated (6), but data describing the use of microcapsules for this purpose have not been reported.

One can envision capsule-packed columns or towers carrying out highly effective liquid/liquid extractions. Since each microcapsule contains a finite volume of liquid, the capsules in a packed column should act as multiple self-contained extractors. A single pass of a feed stream through a capsule-packed tower should yield results equivalent to a multi-stage extraction process. Because the high surface area of microcapsules is permanently fixed by a polymer membrane, one is not concerned with emulsifying two immiscible liquids. One also is not concerned with coalescence of two phases of an emulsion after extraction is complete. If microcapsules could be reversibly charged and discharged, permanent capsule-packed towers capable of carrying out a variety of efficient liquid/liquid extractions could be constructed.

This paper summarizes results of an experimental study designed to explore the validity of the above concepts using recently developed microcapsules with the necessary membrane transport properties (7). All of the extractions reported here involved water-filled microcapsules as packing for a column through which a feed stream of organic solvent solutions of various amines was passed.

## Experimental

Microcapsules containing water were prepared by a patented procedure (7). Capsule size was 300-600µ diameter; water content of the capsules was ~80 wt%. The capsules were isolated by washing with excess pentane and air dried briefly before use. Liquid/liquid extraction experiments were made by loosely packing the water capsules in a chromatographic column (1/2 inch I.D.) to a height of 10-12 inches. The weight of capsules packed for each experiment was recorded. Solutions of monoethanolamine (MEA), triethanolamine (TEA), and triethylenetetramine (TETA) in chloroform ($CHCl_3$) or toluene were then passed through the column by gravity feed from a large reservoir at a constant rate of 5 ml/min. Amine contents of the effluent stream from the column were determined by potentiometric titration with HCl. Such analyses were made on each 50 or 100 ml. aliquot of effluent collected. Results have been plotted as g amine removed by the column as a function of effluent volume. Theoretical curves shown represent the cumulative weight of amine taken from the organic solvent effluent solution for the case of 100% amine removal.

## Results & Discussion

Figure 1 establishes that a column packed with water capsules effectively removes MEA from a chloroform solution. With an initial MEA concentration of 2.0 g/100g $CHCl_3$, 15.4 g of water capsules packed in the column completely removed the MEA from 500 ml of eluted $CHCl_3$ solution. No amine was detected in the effluent stream from the column until the total volume passed through the column exceeded 500 ml. The capsules contained ~80 wt% water, so this is equivalent to ~12.3 g water completely extracting 14 g of MEA from 500 ml of $CHCl_3$ solution. Furthermore, this extraction was accomplished by a single pass through the column. MEA is preferentially soluble in water, but a one-step extraction of MEA dissolved in $CHCl_3$ (10g/ 500 ml) carried out in a separating funnel with 13 g water removed only 75% of the amine from the $CHCl_3$. This demonstrates how much more effectively the same amount of water in a capsule-packed column removes MEA from $CHCl_3$. Once 700 ml of $CHCl_3$ have been passed through the column, the total weight of MEA retained by the column ( ~20 g) remained constant or declined slightly. Thus, 20 g is taken as the

maximum capacity of the column under the specified operation conditions. The effect of flow rate, initial MEA concentration, and
other operating parameters on column performance and maximum capacity of the column has not been examined.

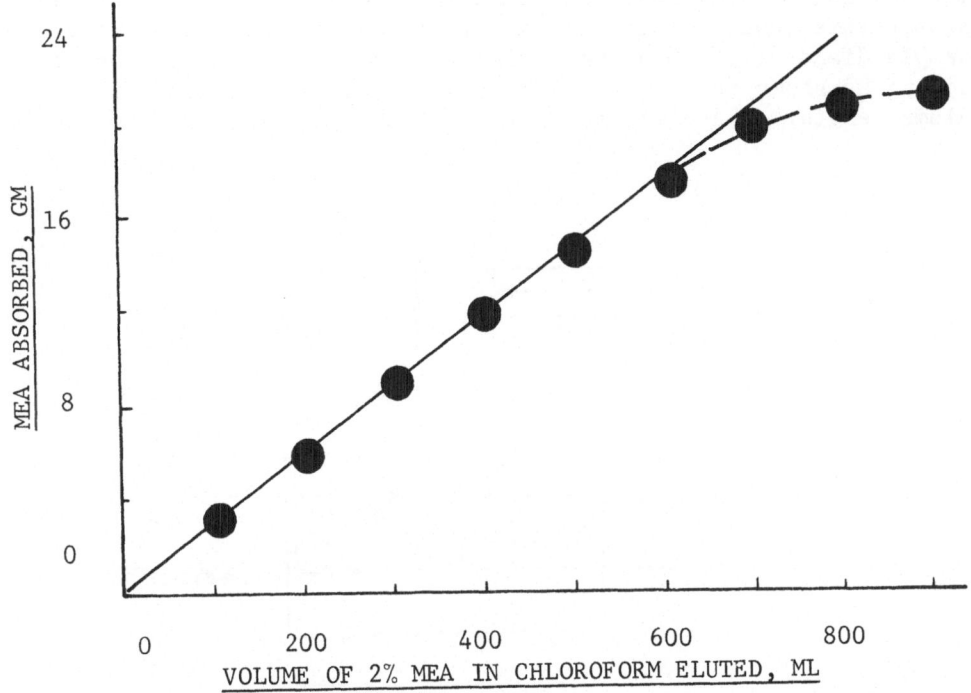

Figure 1:  Elution of MEA from a $CHCl_3$ solution containing 2% MEA
           (W/W) into water capsules at 25°C. Solid line: calculat-
           ed absorption for 100% MEA removal; ●,experimental values.

           Significantly, the data of Figure 1 show that performance of
the capsule-packed column does not begin to deteriorate until one
has reached ∼75% of maximum column capacity. This means the cut-
off point for effective operation of the column is relatively sharp.
The high column capacity and sharp cut-off point for complete MEA
removal are attributed to the ability of each capsule to remove a
finite amount of MEA from the $CHCl_3$ stream. The capsule packing
enables the column to behave as a unique countercurrent extractor.
Figure 2 is a schematic drawing of a capsule-packed column that
illustrates this point. When elution of the $CHCl_3$ solution begins,
those capsules located in the upper region of the column (Zone AB

in Figure 2) cause complete MEA removal from the $CHCl_3$ solution.
Capsules located below point B initially are exposed only to $CHCl_3$,
free of MEA and hence, represent extractors containing fresh extraction fluid. Column length $\ell_{AB}$ represents a finite length of
the column packing and in this length, MEA removal from the $CHCl_3$
is complete. It is postulated that the MEA concentration falls off
exponentially from $C_o$ (2 g/100 g $CHCl_3$) to $C_b = 0$ due to the multiple
liquid/liquid extractions that occur as the $CHCl_3$ solution passes
through this length of column ($\ell_{AB}$). If one assumes an average
capsule diameter of 450µ and envisions a perfect vertical capsule
packing as shown in Figure 2, there would be 22 capsules/cm of
column length. Feed stream passed through such a column would

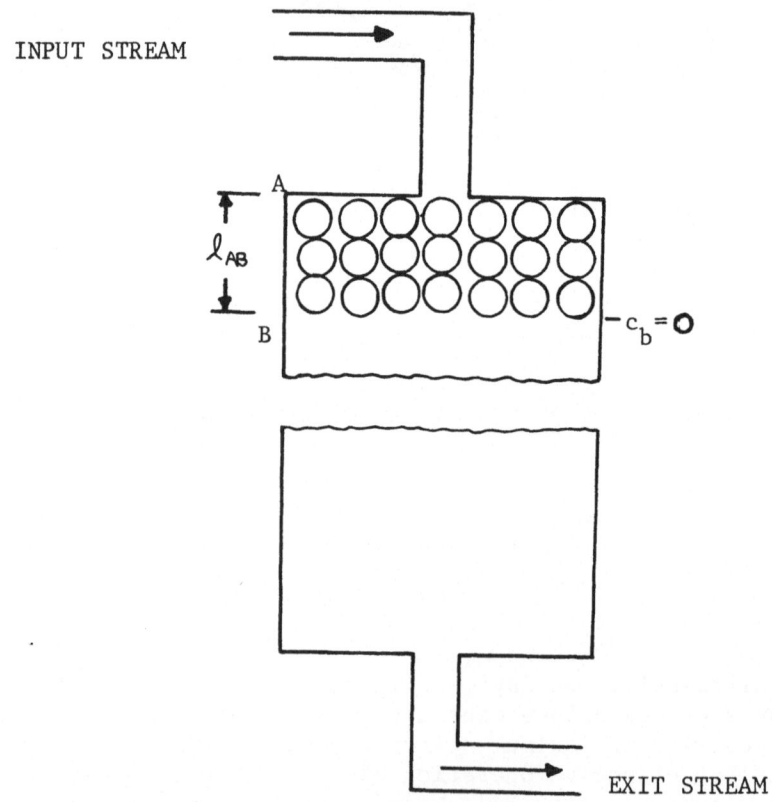

Figure 2:    Schematic drawing of capsule-packed column. Zone AB re-
             presents the finite length of column ($\ell_{AB}$) in which the
             solute concentration of the eluted stream falls from $C_o$
             to $C_b = 0$.

in essence be subjected to 22 countercurrent liquid/liquid extractors per cm of column.    A  randomly packed column may not contain this many extraction stages/cm of column.   Nevertheless, it is repeated exposure to numerous miniature extractors which gives the capsule-packed column such a high degree of effectiveness insofar as MEA removal is concerned.    As elution of the $CHCl_3$ through the column continues, the capsules at point A become effectively "saturated" with MEA under the given flow conditions and hence, this causes point B to begin to slowly move down the column.    Maximum capacity is observed once point A reaches the bottom of the column.

It is relevant to note briefly that transfer of MEA into the water-filled microcapsules occurs through a capsule wall that con-sists of a partially hydrolyzed ethylene-vinyl acetate polymer cross-linked with isocyanate.    This wall is swollen by the $CHCl_3$ solution thereby enabling the observed mass transfer to occur.  For the capsules used in this study, the dry capsule wall thickness is about 18 $\mu$.    The swollen wall thickness was not measured, but equilibrium swelling values in toluene for such capsule walls range from 3 to 5 g toluene/g dry capsule wall.    Whether or not equilibrium exchange of MEA through the swollen capsule walls into the capsule can occur during the eluent's passage through the column has not been estab-lished.    Furthermore, water can diffuse from the capsule into the organic solvent stream.    The raffinate undoubtedly contains water much like it would in the case of a conventional liquid/liquid ex-traction process.

The experiments with MEA were repeated by using a TEA solution in $CHCl_3$ (2 g /100 g $CHCl_3$) as the eluent.  Figure 3 illustrates the effectiveness of the capsule-packed column (15.5 g capsules) insofar as TEA removal is concerned.    In this case, about 8.8. g of TEA have been removed from 300 ml of $CHCl_3$ by ~ 12.3 g of water. Increasing the volume of $CHCl_3$ solution eluted beyond this point led to a steadily decreasing efficiency of TEA removal.  Apparent saturation of the column occurred after 600 ml of eluent had been passed.    The maximum capacity of the column under the specified operating conditions (~16.5 g TEA removed) is only slightly less than that found for MEA.    However, the point at which TEA first appears in the effluent stream falls at ~50% of the column's total TEA capacity (i.e. ~8 g TEA can be removed/12.3 g $H_2O$ with no trace of TEA left in the effluent stream).    These observations probably reflect a lower partition coefficient for TEA between water and $CHCl_3$.    As in the case of MEA, optimum column operating condi-tions were not established.

An experiment with a toluene solution of TETA as eluent (2 g TETA/100 g toluene) was also carried out.  As before, 15.5 g of water capsules were packed in the column.  Figure 4 contains results obtained.    In this case, only ~200 ml of toluene solution were

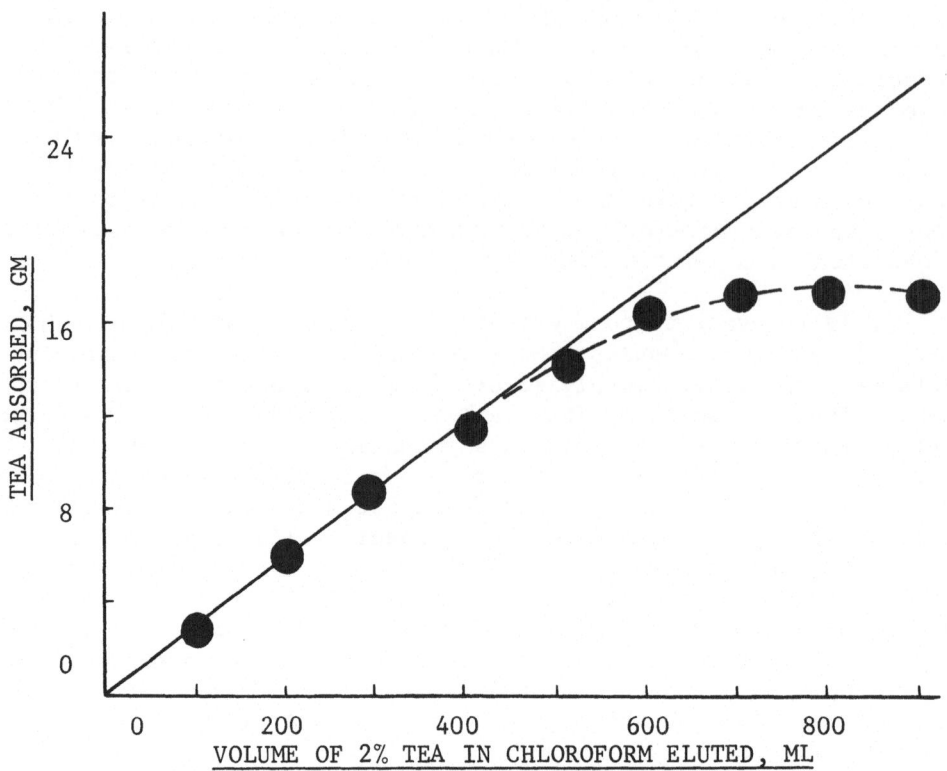

Figure 3:  Elution of TEA from a CHCl$_3$ containing 2% TEA (W/W) into
water capsules at 25°C.  Solid line: Calculated absorption for 100% TEA removal; ●, experimental values.

eluted before TETA began to appear in the eluted toluene stream.The
curve calculated for 100% TETA removal and the experimentally determined curve for TETA removal deviate in a steadily increasing
manner until the column's maximum capacity of~16.5 g TETA is reached.
Thus, the point where TETA retention by the toluene eluent becomes
detectable occurs at ~22% of the maximum capacity of the column
under the specified operation conditions.  That is, only 3.8 g TETA
are absorbed per 12.3 g water before TETA begins to appear in the
eluted stream.

Since reversibility of the extraction  process in a capsule-
packed column is a very desirable feature, the possibility of removing MEA from water capsules has been examined.  This was accomplished by passing 500 ml of 2% MEA in CHCl$_3$ (W/W).

TABLE 1
Effect of cycling on Capsule-Packed Column Performance

| Cycle No. | MEA ABSORBED, %* | MEA Removed, %** | Cumulative wt.of MEA Absorbed, gm |
|-----------|------------------|------------------|-----------------------------------|
| 1 | 100 | 64.4 | 5.2 |
| 2 | 98.2 | 49.7 | 9.8 |
| 3 | 98.8 | 50.0 | 12.1 |
| 4 | 95.3 | 46.6 | 13.9 |
| 5 | 98.2 | 41.2 | 16.6 |
| 6 | 96.8 | 36.5 | 19.9 |

* % of MEA in 500 ml $CH1_3$ eluent absorbed by the capsule-packed column.

** % of MEA in capsule-packed column removed by 200 ml water wash.

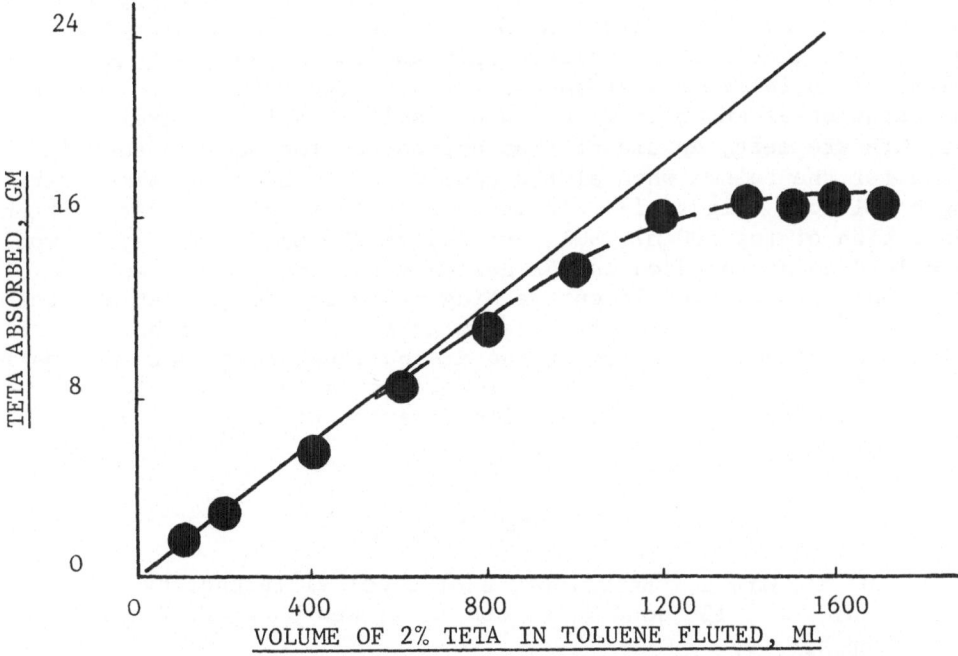

Figure 4: Elution of TETA from a toluene solution containing 2% TETA (W/W) into water capsules at $25^{\circ}C$. Solid line: calculated absorption for 100% TETA removal; ●, experimental values.

over 15.5 g water capsules and monitoring the weight of MEA transferred to the capsules. After this, 200 ml of distilled water were
eluted through the same capsule-packed column and the weight of MEA
extracted from the capsules by the water wash was determined. This
$CHCl_3$ extraction/water wash cycle was repeated a total of 6 times.
Table I summarizes results obtained. The first column is the cycle
number. The second column is the percent of the MEA in 500 ml $CHCl_3$
absorbed by the capsules in each cycle. The third column is the percent of the MEA in the capsule-packed column removed in each cycle by
the 200 ml water wash. The fourth column is the weight of MEA left
in the capsule-packed column after each $CHCl_3$ extraction/water wash
cycle.

As shown in Table I, the first extraction step led to 100% MEA
removal from 500 ml $CHCl_3$. The first water wash removed only 64.0%
of this MEA from the capsules thereby leaving 5.2 g MEA in the capsules. During the second cycle, 98% of the MEA in 500 ml of $CHCl_3$
was extracted by the capsule packing, whereas the subsequent water
wash removed only 50% of the MEA in the capsules. This leads to a
net increase in the MEA content of the capsules. The $CHCl_3$ extrac-
tion/water wash cycle was repeated four more times. In each case,
95-99% of the MEA in the $CHCl_3$ solution eluted over the capsules
is removed. As shown in column 3 of Table I, the accompanying water
wash cycles consistently removed only 40-50% of the MEA in the capsules. This leads to a steady increase in the weight of MEA left in
the capsules as shown in column 4 of Table I. After 6 cycles, ~20
g of MEA are left, an amount that approaches the maximum capacity
found for the column when eluted continuously under the same operating conditions (Figure 1). It is reasonable to expect that continued
repetition of the 500 ml $CHCl_3$ extraction/200 ml $H_2O$ washcycle would
soon lead to a breakdown in the column's ability to separate MEA
from $CHCl_3$. A more efficient washing procedure (e.g., replace the
water with an acidic alcohol/water mixture) may prevent buildup of
MEA in the column. In spite of the MEA buildup, these data demonstrate
the ability of capsules to be at least partially regenerated when
used as a packed bed for liquid/liquid extractions.

## References

1.  J. A. Herbig, "Encyclopedia of Chemical Technology", 2nd
    Ed., Vol. 13, John Wiley and Sons, New York, N. Y., 1967,
    pp 436-456.

2.  C. E. Anderson, Et. al., "Microencapsulation", MIR
    Management Reports, Boston, Massachusetts, 1963.

3.  T.M.S. Chang, "Artifical Cells", C.C. Thomas, Publishers,
    Springfield, Illinois, 1972.

4.  R. E. Sparks, N. S. Mason, M. H. Litt, P.M. Meier, and O.
    Lindan, Trans. Am. Soc. Artif. Internal Organ XVII, 229
    (1971).

5.  M. Morishita, M. Fukushima, and Y. Inaba, Div. Org.
    Coatings and Plastics Chem. Preprints 33(2) 603 (1973).

6.  N. N. Li, AICHE Journal 17, 459 (1971).

7.  R. Bayless, C. Shank, R. Botham, and D. Werkmeister,
    U. S. Patent 3,674,704 (1972).

# LIQUID-CRYSTAL CONTAINING LIGHT SENSITIVE MICROCAPSULES

Souichi KUBO

Department of Photographic Engineering
Chiba University
33-1 Yayoicho, Chiba City
Chiba, Japan

This paper describes an experimental method of making cholesteric liquid-crystal containing microcapsules of complex hydrophilic colloid materials as well as a photographic application. The purpose of this study is to obtain a colored photographic image whose tonal characteristics are a function of temperature.

## I. METHOD OF MAKING MICROCAPSULES

In our preferred method of making microcapsules, the colloid material deposits around each liquid crystal droplet forming a dense oil-impervious casing with the liquid crystal nucleus at the center. In this experiment, gelatin and gum arabic were used as colloid materials and a mixture of cholesteric liquid crystals diluted with chloroform was used as the nucleus. The complex co-acervation process was applied to encapsulate. The details of this experiment are shown in the following Tables.

MIXED CHOLESTERIC LIQUID-CRYSTALS USED IN THIS EXPERIMENT

The following composition is expressed by weight.

$$
\begin{array}{lcr}
\text{cholesteryl nonanoate} & \text{---} & 60\% \\
\text{cholesteryl oleyl carbonate} & \text{---} & 4\% \\
\text{cholesteryl butyrate} & \text{---} & 16\% \\
\text{cholesteryl linolate} & \text{---} & 20\% \\
\end{array}
$$
(operating range --- $20^{\circ}C \sim 30^{\circ}C$)

The above weight proportion of mixed cholesteric liquid-crystals for dilution in chloroform was chosen for more distinctive coloration. Other combinations may be used also.

COLLOID MATERIALS USED IN THIS EXPERIMENT

Polycation --- Gelatin, Nitta type P, Batch No. 1762
               Iso-electric point --- pH 5.4
               (photographic grade gelatin)
Polyanion  --- Gum arabic

PROCESS OF MAKING MICROCAPSULES

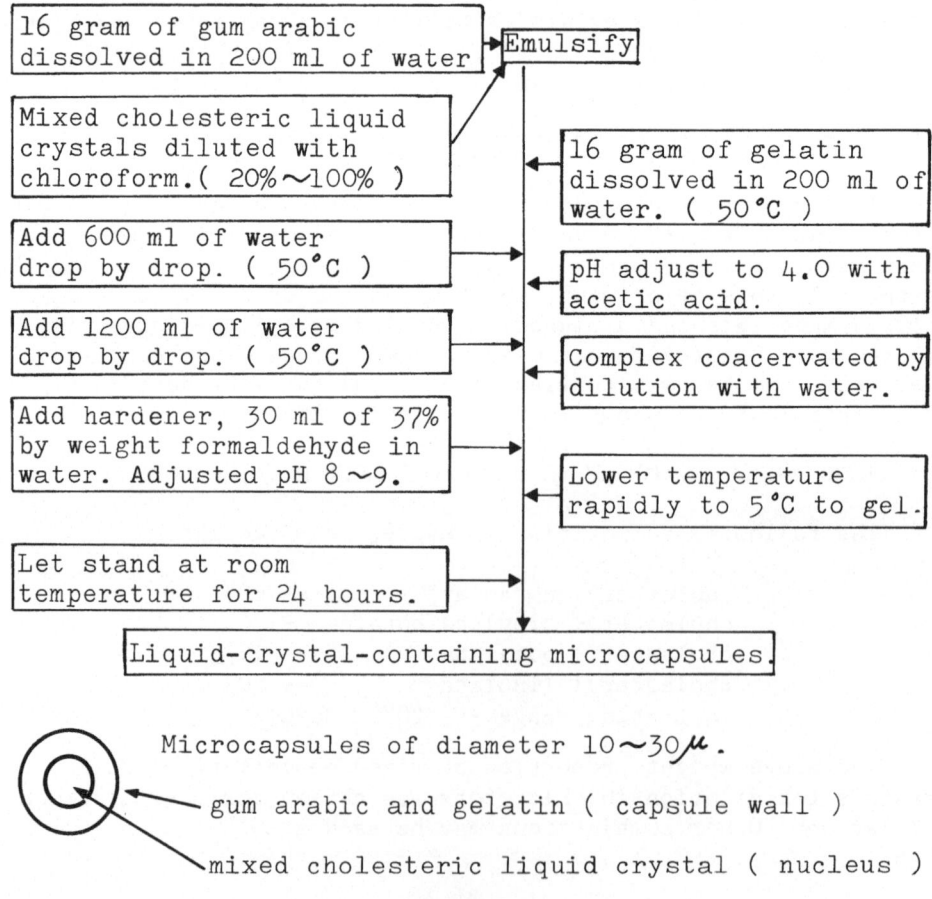

| 16 gram of gum arabic dissolved in 200 ml of water | → | Emulsify |

Mixed cholesteric liquid crystals diluted with chloroform.( 20%~100% )

16 gram of gelatin dissolved in 200 ml of water. ( 50°C )

Add 600 ml of water drop by drop. ( 50°C )

pH adjust to 4.0 with acetic acid.

Add 1200 ml of water drop by drop. ( 50°C )

Complex coacervated by dilution with water.

Add hardener, 30 ml of 37% by weight formaldehyde in water. Adjusted pH 8~9.

Lower temperature rapidly to 5°C to gel.

Let stand at room temperature for 24 hours.

Liquid-crystal-containing microcapsules.

Microcapsules of diameter 10~30μ.

gum arabic and gelatin ( capsule wall )

mixed cholesteric liquid crystal ( nucleus )

Figure 1

COLORATION OF MIXED-LIQUID-CRYSTALS CONTAINING MICROCAPSULES

   The mixed cholesteric liquid-crystals containing microcapsules
were coated onto a black surfaced support with a binder (in this
case a solution of 2% gelatin in water was used).  After the coating was dried, the colors of the microcapsules were measured by
means of photographic photometry.  The microcapsules containing
the mixed cholesteric liquid-crystals diluted with 30% of chloroform by weight showed the sharpest coloration.  The results are
shown in the next figure.

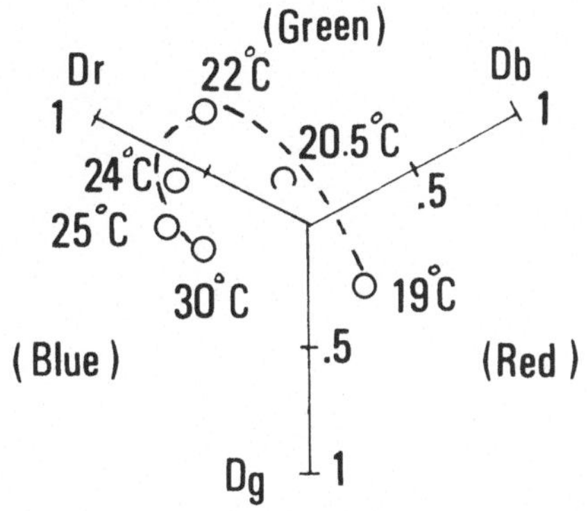

Figure 2

   Here the optical densities for the three basic colors, red,
green and blue are plotted on three 120 degree axes.  Therefore
the sector opposite a specific color axis is the area of the
greatest reflection of that color.  Hence we see that $19^{\circ}$C the
reflection is entirely in the red region which at higher temperatures shifts to the green and then to the blue region.

   Since the color of a liquid-crystal coating depends also on
the viewing angle one would expect multiple colors in the reflection from the curved surfaces of the microcapsules.  The fact that
this does not happen is undoubtedly due to the fact that the microcapsules flatten after being coated onto the substrate.  This
flattening is caused by loss of chloroform through evaporation
from the nucleus of the capsules.

   These microcapsules should find interesting uses in printing
inks.

II.  METHOD OF MAKING LIGHT SENSITIVE MICROCAPSULES CONTAINING
     MIXED CHOLESTERIC LIQUID CRYSTALS

   In the microcapsules produced by this experiment, the capsule walls contain a gelatino-silver-halide photographic emulsion in which color-couplers are incorporated beforehand.

PHOTOGRAPHIC EMULSION USED IN THIS EXPERIMENT

A general formula of chlorobromide emulsion was selected. The gelatin in this photographic emulsion is the same gelatin as used in the previous microcapsulation.

COLOR-COUPLER

The following type of color-coupler was used in this experiment.

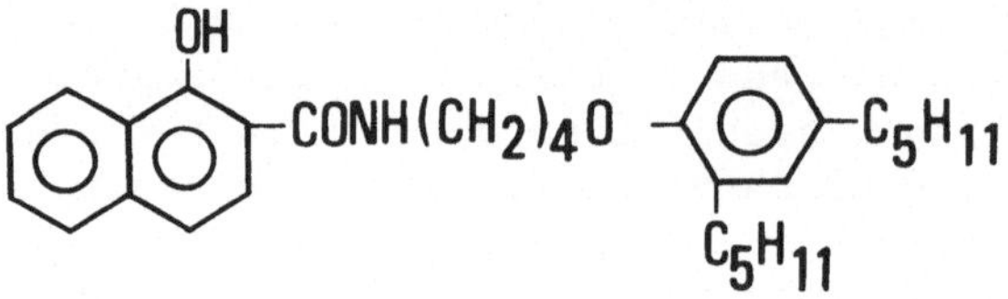

1-hydroxy-2-[$\delta$(2,4-di-tert.amylphenoxy)-n-butyl] -naphthamide

Figure 3

## PROCESS OF MAKING LIGHT SENSITIVE MICROCAPSULES

Detail of the process is shown in text.

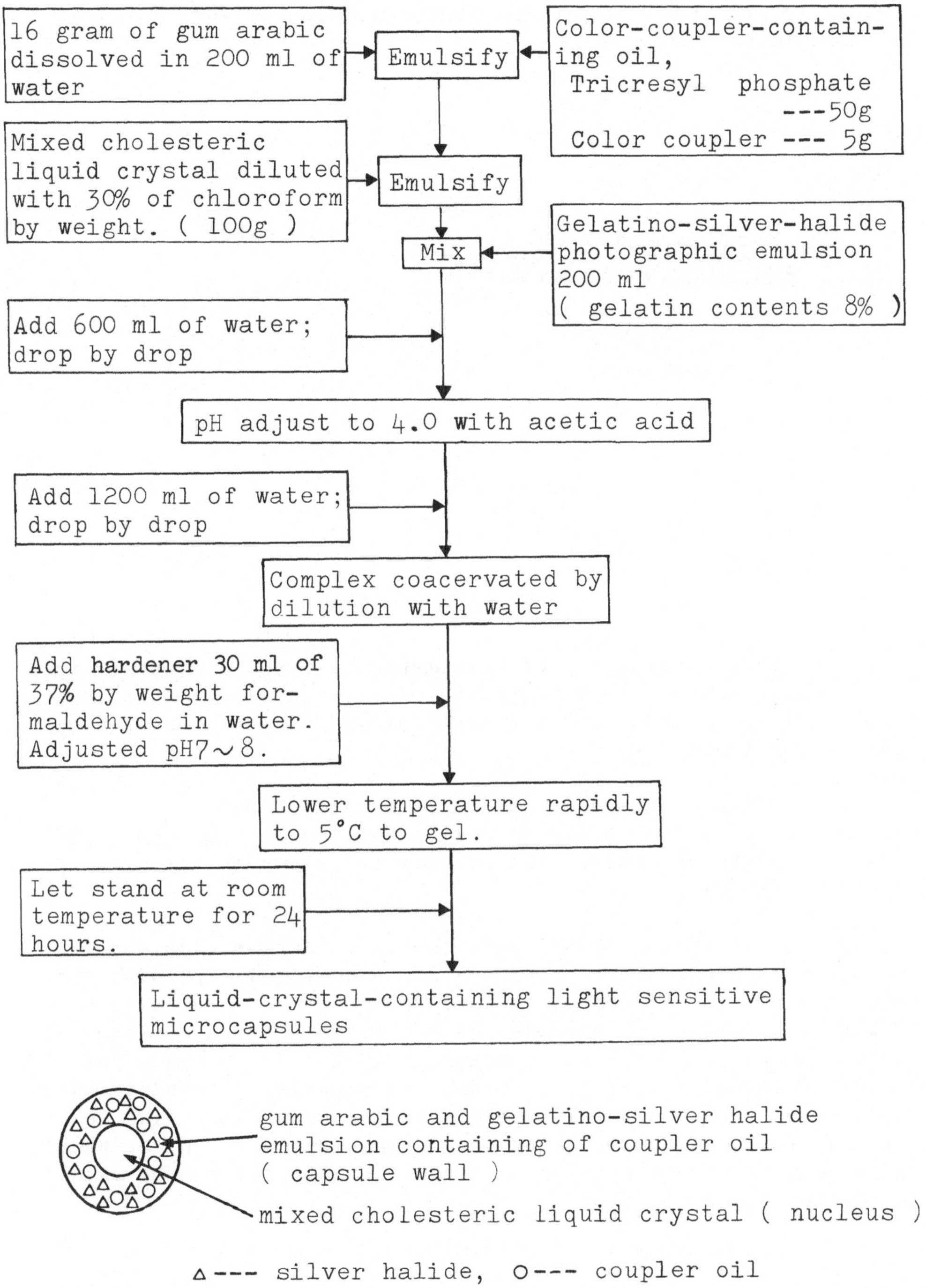

| | | |
|---|---|---|
| 16 gram of gum arabic dissolved in 200 ml of water | → Emulsify ← | Color-coupler-containing oil, Tricresyl phosphate ---50g Color coupler --- 5g |

| | | |
|---|---|---|
| Mixed cholesteric liquid crystal diluted with 30% of chloroform by weight. ( 100g ) | → Emulsify | |

Mix ← Gelatino-silver-halide photographic emulsion 200 ml ( gelatin contents 8% )

Add 600 ml of water; drop by drop →

pH adjust to 4.0 with acetic acid

Add 1200 ml of water; drop by drop →

Complex coacervated by dilution with water

Add hardener 30 ml of 37% by weight formaldehyde in water. Adjusted pH7∼8. →

Lower temperature rapidly to 5°C to gel.

Let stand at room temperature for 24 hours. →

Liquid-crystal-containing light sensitive microcapsules

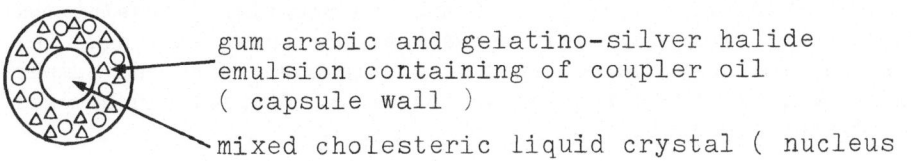

gum arabic and gelatino-silver halide emulsion containing of coupler oil ( capsule wall )

mixed cholesteric liquid crystal ( nucleus )

△--- silver halide,  ○--- coupler oil

Figure 4

LIQUID-CRYSTAL CONTAINING PHOTOGRAPHIC MATERIAL

   The new type of photographic material containing of liquid
crystal is produced.  The cross-sectional view of this material
is shown in the next.

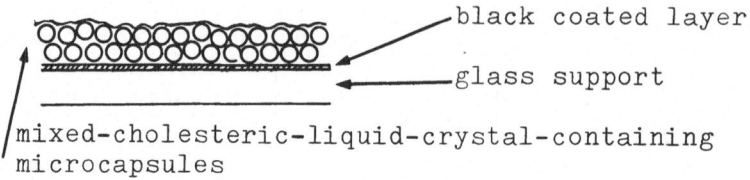

                            black coated layer

                            glass support

mixed-cholesteric-liquid-crystal-containing
microcapsules

Figure 5

   The light sensitivity of this material is of a moderate speed
and is equivalent to a photographic paper.  This photographic
material is used as a printing material and can be processed by
Kodak C chemicals.

   For this photographic material, the variation of color
differences between the images and background depends upon the
variation of temperature.  The results are shown in the next
figure.

   As can be seen in the figure the image intensities Db-Di
(Db --- background density, Di --- image density) vary with the
temperature.  If the images on this photographic material are
viewed or photographed through the red filter, as an example, the
maximum image intensity is observed at 22°C.  In the same way, the
minimum image intensity at 24°C and the negative intensity maximum
at 30°C are observed.  This means that the phase of images is
changed from positive to negative continuously with the temperature
variation.  This new type of photographic material can be used for
temperature recording.

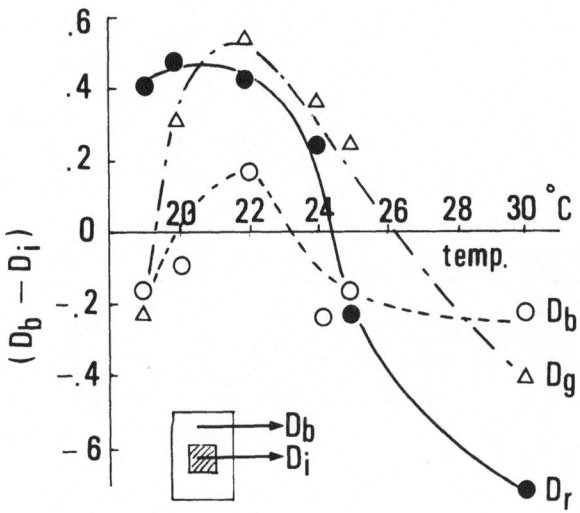

Dr --- Red filter density, measured through
       wratten No.92.
Dg --- Green filter density, measured through
       wratten No.93.
Db --- Blue filter density, measured through
       wratten No.94.


Figure 6

# MICROENCAPSULATED PESTICIDES

C. B. DeSavigny & E. E. Ivy

Agchem-Decco Division / Pennwalt Corporation

P. O. Box 3608 / Bryan, Texas   77801

As DDT and other chlorinated hydrocarbons are being phased out because of their long persistence in the environment, the use of certain organophosphate insecticides is increasing substantially.  The latter, however, have the disadvantages of high toxicity and too limited persistence.  They are degraded in the environment so rapidly that frequent applications, which tend to be put on at excessively high dosages, are necessary. This is an inherently wasteful, expensive, and at times, hazardous practice.  We have shown that microencapsulation of these insecticides prolongs their efficacy sufficiently to allow the number and rate of required applications to be reduced.  Simultaneously, oral and dermal tests with laboratory animals indicate a significantly reduced mammalian toxicity for microencapsulated insecticides.

## MICROENCAPSULATION PROCESS

The concept of microencapsulation has been known for many years, and many techniques are described in the patent literature (1).  This paper is limited to a procedure which has proved effective in the microencapsulation of pesticides by formation of a polymer skin around a liquid which has been dispersed into fine droplets.  The resulting microspheres each contain some of the liquid pesticide.  The procedure, which has been described in detail elsewhere (2), involves dispersing in an aqueous medium, by means of high speed agitation, a liquid pesticide containing a dissolved monomer.  Following dispersion of the organic phase, interfacial polymerization at the droplet surface is carried out by the addition of a second, water soluble, monomer to the continuous aqueous phase. The resulting pesticide-containing capsules can then be recovered as a dry powder or left as a water slurry. Variations important to the performance of the products are achieved by controlling the following parameters.

1. Polymer composition of capsule wall. The choice of monomers can be varied to produce any of several interfacial polycondensation products as wall materials, such as polyamides, polyesters, polyureas, polyurethanes, and polycarbonates. A range of polymers is available within each of these categories, again depending on choice of monomers. It is also possible to vary wall composition by forming copolymers by the simple process of using a mixture of oil soluble or of water soluble monomers.

2. Degree of crosslinking. In those instances where it is essential to have a higher degree of wall integrity than that obtained with these straight chain polymers, it is possible to crosslink the wall polymers.

3. Capsule wall thickness. Thickness of capsule wall is a function of concentration of the oil soluble monomer (or monomers). Since an excess of the water soluble monomer is normally used, the reaction continues thickening the wall until all of the oil soluble monomers are consumed.

4. Capsule size. The size of capsules is determined by the degree of agitation and by the type of emulsifying agent used in the continuous phase. Capsule size can be varied from an average diameter of a few microns to a millimeter. There is, of course, a range of sizes obtained. For example, an average capsule size of 70 microns corresponds to a Gaussian distribution with capsule sizes ranging from 20 to 150 microns.

5. Physical form of product. The final product can be left as a water slurry or the capsules can be filtered, washed, and dried to a free-flowing powder. A water slurry has been found extremely useful in the pesticide area, for in addition to being more economical to manufacture, it need only be diluted with water in order to be ready for field application as a sprayable product.

6. Additives. Many additives, such as U.V. light absorbers, antioxidants, and synergists, may be dissolved in the oil phase being encapsulated. These additives, of course, need to be soluble in the oil and not reactive with the monomers.

Materials which can be encapsulated are liquids, solutions, melts, or suspensions of fine powders. A limiting factor for the encapsulation process as described is that the encapsulate must be insoluble in water. It is possible, however, to reverse the procedure to overcome this. An aqueous solution of the water soluble monomer can be dispersed in an oil. The oil-soluble monomer is then added to the continuous oil phase. In this case the encapsulated product can be left as an oil slurry or worked up to a dry powder.

A second process limitation is that the material being encapsulated should not react with polymerization monomers. It has been possible in some cases to work around this limitation. Encapsulation of diamines, for instance, can be carried out by allowing part of the amine itself to act as a monomer. In some cases, the reactive group in the encapsulate may be sterically hindered enough that the desired polymerization reaction takes place preferentially.

## PROPERTIES OF CAPSULES AND ENCAPSULATED METHYL PARATHION

One type of wall material, a polyamide with a polyurea crosslinking network, has been used to encapsulate xylene as a free-flowing dry powder. These capsules were found to hold their contents tenaciously, losing only about one per cent per day in an open dish at 50 degrees C or under a pressure of 0.1 mm Hg at room temperature. Figure I shows a series of photographs of these capsules taken with an electron scanning microscope. The surface appears to be very rough and extremely porous. High magnification photographs of capsules containing other materials differ in appearance. This fact supports observations that each encapsulation system is unique and generalities are difficult to make.

There are several ways in which an encapsulated material can be released from its shell. It can diffuse through the wall, or it can be leached out by water or other solvent. The capsules can be broken by an application of pressure from the outside (crushing) or a pressure build up on the inside (bursting). Wall degradation is a possibility with some formulations but unlikely when the wall has been crosslinked.

This encapsulation process has been applied to methyl parathion (O,O-dimethyl-O-p-nitrophenyl phosphorothioate), a commonly used insecticide. In its conventional formulation as an emulsifiable concentrate (E.C.), methyl parathion has low persistence ranging from a few hours to several days. It also has a very high mammalian toxicity. For example, the oral $LD_{50}$ is 10 mg/kg for white mice (3). Encapsulated methyl parathion is about one-tenth as toxic with an average oral $LD_{50}$ of 100 mg/kg. The dermal $LD_{50}$ in albino rabbits is less

FULL CAPSULES

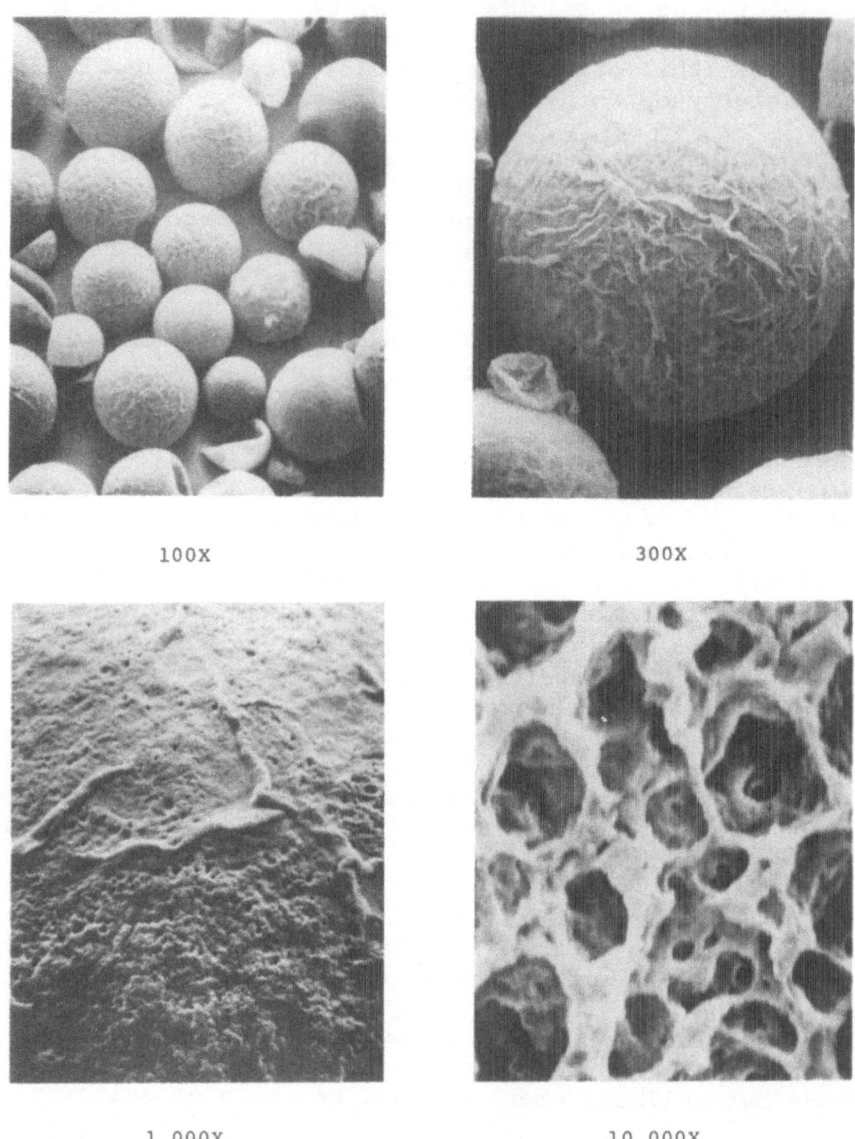

100X                                    300X

1,000X                                  10,000X

Courtesy of Dr. John Meakin, Research Laboratories, The Franklin
Institute, Philadelphia, Pennsylvania.

Figure I

than 100 mg/kg for methyl parathion E.C., whereas it is greater than 1200 mg/kg for the encapsulated material. These toxicity data were calculated on the basis of active ingredient present.

Pencap$^{TM}$ M is the Pennwalt trademark for an aqueous suspension of encapsulated methyl parathion. It may be applied with ordinary ground or air equipment. After application of the material, the water evaporates and controlled release of methyl parathion occurs through the porous walls of the capsules. Comparisons of insecticidal effectiveness of encapsulated methyl parathion against standard formulations of emulsifiable concentrate have been made both in the laboratory and in the field against the following insects:

| Insect | Host |
| --- | --- |
| Bollworm | Cotton foliage |
| Boll weevil | Cotton foliage |
| Cricket | Bean foliage |
| Two-spot mite | Apple and bean foliage |
| Tomato fruitworm | Tomato fruit |
| Corn earworm | Sweet corn |
| Japanese beetle | Bean foliage |
| Gypsy moth | Oak foliage |

The results showed a definite increase in insect control for a longer period of time for the encapsulated methyl parathion versus standard formulations. Examples of tests and results follow.

Bean plants were sprayed with encapsulated and E.C. methyl parathion formulations using Tee JET 6510 nozzles. Leaves were harvested randomly at various intervals and assayed in the laboratory using crickets (Gyryllus domesticus). Six leaves and ten crickets were placed in each jar. Kill was recorded after 48 hours. Similar tests were conducted using Japanese beetles. At 0.50 lb active per acre (0.56 kg/ha), 100% of both insects were killed after five days and 40-80% after eight days with the encapsulated material. The E.C. was completely ineffective after three days for crickets and after five days for Japanese beetles.

Samples of encapsulated methyl parathion, prepared with various degrees of crosslinking in the wall, were sprayed on cotton plants. Infestations at intervals with boll weevils or bollworms showed that the degree of crosslinking present in the capsule wall has a significant effect on the rate of release. An optimum degree of crosslinking was 25% with a polyamide-polyurea wall composition. The preparation showed 100% control of bollworms after seven days and 72% after eleven days.

Methyl parathion E.C. gave only 60% control after three days and 16% after five days. The rate of application was one pound per acre (1.1 kg/ha).

Encapsulation has had a second significant and unexpected effect on pesticides, i.e., a lower dosage of active material is required for equal control. In one test, boll weevils were placed on cotton leaves sprayed seven days previously. Foliage which had been sprayed with methyl parathion E.C. at a dosage of 0.25 lb/acre (0.28 kg/ha) produced no weevil mortality. Foliage sprayed with encapsulated methyl parathion at 0.10 lb/acre (0.11 kg/ha) resulted in 74% mortality.

This microencapsulation technique is applicable to many pesticidal compounds, and investigation of this process with additional materials is continuing.

## REFERENCES

1.  M. W. Ranney, Microencapsulation Technology (Noyes Development Corporation, Park Ridge, N.J., 1969).

2.  U. S. Patent 3,577,515, Jan E. Vandegaer to Pennwalt Corporation.

3.  Toxicological data supplied by Pharmacology Research Inc., Darby, Pennsylvania.

ARTIFICIAL CELLS AND MICROCAPSULES:    COMPARISION OF STRUCTURAL

AND FUNCTIONAL DIFFERENCES

T. M. S. Chang

Professor of Physiology, Faculty of Medicine
McGill University
Montreal, P.Q., Canada

The industrial microcapsules first disclosed in the patent
literature in 1957 are prepared as microscopic containers of oily
material (1).  These microcapsules containing oil are coated on
paper.  Mechanical pressure rupture these microcapsules, releasing
their oily content to form prints - the basis of the well-known
NCR carbonless paper.  Since then, most of the industrial and
pharmaceutical microencapsulation  technology are similarly
prepared to contain medication,  fuel, perfumes, adhesives, and
others.  In all cases, the enclosing wall of these microcapsules
are made as impermeable to external and internal molecules as
possible, and the enclosed material can act only when the microcapsule wall is disrupted releasing the enclosed material.  The
enclosing walls are, therefore, rather thick (greater than 1
micron).

The artificial cells first reported in 1957 (2-5) differ from
these industrial microcapsules in a number of important points.
In artificial cells, the contents are aqueous solution or suspension of biologically active material like enzymes, proteins,
and detoxicants.  The enclosed material do not depend on being
released from the enclosing membrane for action.  While remaining
at all times enveloped by the enclosing membrane and prevented
from coming into direct contact with the external environment, the
enclosed materials act on external permeant molecules diffusing
into the artificial cells.  The enclosing membrane of artificial
cells is prepared in such a way that while impermeable to macro-
molecules or suspensions, it is extremely permeable to most of the
solutes normally present in the biological fluid.  This high
permeability is a result of the ultrathin membrane  (0.05 micron)
and porosity ( equivalent pore radius of 18° of the artificial cells.

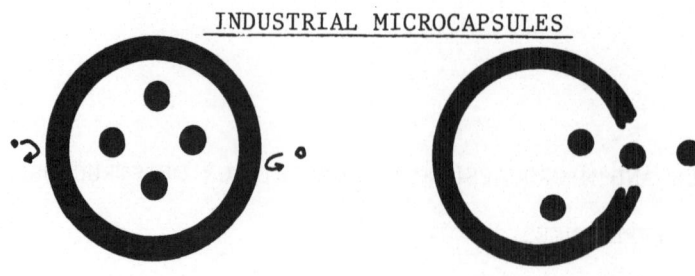

INDUSTRIAL MICROCAPSULES

intact – not functioning                          release
                                          material to function

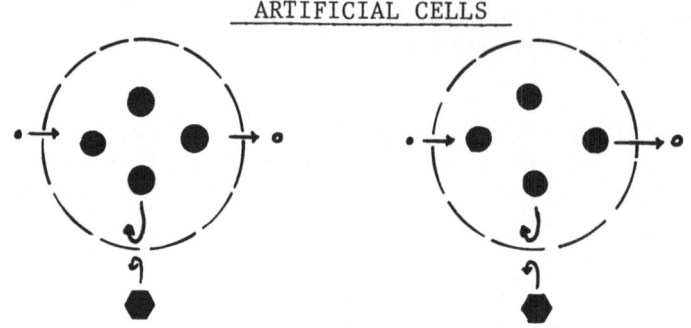

ARTIFICIAL CELLS

functioning while intact

● – enzyme or detoxicant

• – substrates or toxin

o – products of enzyme reaction

⬡ – antibodies or other cells

     As other laboratories became interested in the area of art-
ificial cells and started explorations into this area (25-32),
attempts have been made to make use of the available industrial
microencapsulation technology for the preparation of artificial
cells.  As a result, the initial completely separated interests
in the fields of research in artificial cells and microcapsules
now rapidly merges.  Furthermore, for want of a better word, semipermeable microcapsules have been used to describe these artificial
cells.

The most efficient type of separation can be found in nature
in the form of biological cells. Each biological cell has a
diameter of about 10 microns, with a cell membrane of about 0.01
micron in thickness. This means that the total membrane area
available for diffusion can be extremely large in comparison to the
volume, and that the cell membrane can also be very thin without
loss of mechanical strength. In addition, rapid mixing is possible within the individual microscopic compartments. Biological
cells have very complex and selective enzyme systems to act on
molecules entering the cells. Artificial cells have been prepared
in this laboratory with some of these properties (2-5). Details
can be referred to in the reviews given in the references. The
ultrathin membrane (less than 0.05 micron) and the total surface
area ($2M^2$) is such that the transport rate of 10 ml of 20 micron
diameter artificial cells is 200 times higher than the transport
rate of a standard artificial kidney machine. (Table 1). The
rate of equilibration of solutes across artificial cells would
become obvious in the example of the half-time for equilibration
of only 4.3 seconds for urea for artificial cells of 210.9 micron
diameter.

Solute - T 1/2for Equilibration (210.9 micron diameter)
                                        (seconds)
tritiated water ......................... less than 1.0
urea ....................................... 4.5
creatinine ................................. 17.5
uric acid .................................. 42.5
creatine ................................... 16.6
glucose .................................... 26.2
sucrose .................................... 35.5

There are many variations in using artificial cells in separation (6). The artificial cells can be used to separate a
solute on the basis of size, lipid coefficient and charge. They
can also be used in combination with adsorbent to selectively
remove select molecules which can be adsorbed; in combination with
enzyme in the microcapsules to selectively act on permeant substrate; and in an even more complex system containing a combination of enzyme and adsorbent. Experiments have been carried out
here to study the use of the artificial cell system to separate
small molecules from protein in an in vitro situation, or the use
of a column of artificial cells to separate large molecules from
small molecules (6). Artificial cells containing enzymes have
also been used for in vitro, and also for in vivo use when injected into animals to selectively remove certain substrates (3,5).

For example, artificial cells containing urease injected into
experimental animals selectively converts body urea into ammonia
(3,5,6,). Artificial cells containing urease in an extracorporeal
shunt chamber selectively converts blood urea into ammonia which
can then be removed by ammonia adsorbents (5,8). Artificial cells

TABLE 1

|  | Membrane Area $M^2$ | Membrane Thickness (micron) | Transport Rate- Ratio |
|---|---|---|---|
| MICROCAPSULES Vol: 10 ml Diameter:20 microns | 2 | 0.02 | 1000 |
| MICROCAPSULES Vol: 300 ml Diameter: 2-5 mm | 2 | 0.05 | 200 |
| HEMODIALYSERS (Coil, Plate, or capillary) | 1 | 5.00 | 1 |

containing catalase injected into animals with a congenital de-
ficiency in the enzyme catalase efficiently replaces the deficient
enzyme in selectively removing toxic peroxides from the body (5,9).
Artificial cells containing asparaginase injected into animals can
selectively remove asparagine, thus suppressing the growth of
asparagine-dependent tumours (5,10,11). Artificial cells containing lactase can be used to remove lactose from milk for patients
with a intolerance to milk because of lactase-deficiency. Enzymes
in artificial cells prevented from giving rise to immunological
and hypersensitivity reactions, continue to act efficiently to
remove one selected substrate in the extremely complex biological
fluid, thus giving a highly selective separation system (5,13,14).
The enzymes enclosed within artificial cells are also more stable
when compared to enzymes in free solution (12).

One of the applications of artificial cells has been in the
use of the system in the development of a microcapsule artificial
kidney (5,8, 15-24). Very briefly, the basic principle is as
follows:  300 ml of very large artificial cells (3-5 mm diameter)
packed in a column have a total membrane area of 2.25 $M^2$ - double
the area of a standard artificial kidney (1 $M^2$). The membrane of
each artificial cell is less than 0.05 micron, at least 100 times
thinner than the hemodialysis membrane. The combination of ultrathin membrane and large surface area would result in a potential
transport rate of at least 200 times higher than the standard hemo-
dialyser. By putting adsorbent such as activated charcoal inside

artificial cells uremic toxins can equilibrate rapidly into the artificial cells to be removed by the activated charcoal. The microencapsulated activated charcoal is prevented by microencapsulation from embolising and from adversely affecting the formed elements of blood. Blood compatibility can be achieved by heparinisation of the membrane (16-17) or coating with human albumin (5,15,18,19). Efficiency of removal of uremic metabolites, as expressed by clearance, especially the important large molecules is many times greater for a 300 gm microcapsule artificial kidney (18-22). In this way patients treated for 2 hours on the microcapsule artificial kidney remain as well as patients treated on the large hemodialysis machine for 6-10 hours. At present the removal of water and electrolytes has to be carried out separately. The detailed experimental and clinical results of these studies have already been published (5, 18-22).

The microcapsule artificial kidney has also been used in experiments in animals and for the treatment of patients with acute intoxication (5,15,23,24). Glutethemide (Doriden), methaqualone (Qualone), methyprylon (Noludar), and phenobarbital are removed efficiently in overdosed patients by the microcapsule artificial kidney.

Recently (14) studies have been carried out here to combine the use of artificial cells with synthetic capillary fibres. The results obtained in this study demonstrated the feasibility of using this as the basis of the construction of artificial organs involved in metabolite control.

## REFERENCES

1. Green, B.K. and Schneidcher, L. Microcapsules and Hydrophobic Contents, U.S. Patents, 2,800,457; 2,800,458 (1957)

2. Chang, T.M.S. Hemoglobin Corpuscles, Report of Research Project, B.Sc. Honours, Physiology, McGill University (1957) Montreal, Quebec.

3. Chang, T.M.S. Semipermeable aqueous microcapsules. Science, 146:524, 1964.

4. Chang, T.M.S., MacIntosh, F.C., and Mason, S.G. Semipermeable aqueous microcapsules. Canad. J. Physiol. Pharmacol., 44:115 1966.

5.    Chang, T.M.S.  Artificial Cells.  Charles C. Thomas, Publisher
      Springfield, Illinois, 1972.

6.    Chang, T.M.S.  A new approach to separation using semiper-
      meable microcapsules (artificial cells): combined dialysis,
      catalysis and adsorption.  In Recent developments in Separ-
      ation Science, (ed.) N. Li, Chemical Rubber Co. Cleveland,
      Ohio, 1972.

7.    Chang, T.M.S., and MacIntosh, F.C. (1964), Semipermeable
      aqueous microcapsules, Pharmacologist, 6:198.

8.    Chang, T.M.S.  Semipermeable aqueous microcapsules ("Art-
      ificial cells") with emphasis on experiments in an extra-
      corporeal shunt system. Trans. Amer. Soc. Artif. Int. Organs,
      12:13, 1966.

9.    Chang, T.M.S. and Poznansky, M.J.  Semipermeable microcapsules
      containing catalase for enxyme replacement in acatalasemic
      mice.  Nature, 218:243, 1968.

10.   Chang, T.M.S.  The in vivo effects of semipermeable micro-
      capsules containing L-Asparaginase on 6C3HED lmyphosarcoma.
      Nature, 229:117, 1971.

11.   Chang, T.M.S.  L-Asparaginase Immobilised within Semipermeable
      Microcapsules: in vitro and in vivo stability.  Enzyme
      Journal 14:95, 1973.

12.   Chang, T.M.S.  Stabilisation of enzymes by microencapsula-
      tion with a concentrated protein solution or by microen-
      capsulation followed by cross-linking with gluteraldehyde.
      Biochem. & Biophys. Res. Com. 44:1531, 1971.

13.   Chang, T.M.S. In vitro and in vivo kinetics of enzymes im-
      mobilized by microencapsulation.  Biotechnol. & Bioeng. Symp.,
      3:395, 1972.

14.   Chang, T.M.S.  Biomedical Applications of Artificial Cells.
      Biomedical Engineering 8:334, 1973.

15.   Chang, T.M.S.  Removal of endogenous and exogenous and exo-
      genous toxins by a microencapsulated adsorbent.  Canad. J.
      Physiol. Pharmacol., 47:1043, 1969.

16. Chang, T.M.S., Johnson, L.J., and Ransome,O. (1967): Semipermeable aqueous microcapsules: Nonthrombogenic microcapsules with heparincomplexed membranes. Canad. J. Physiol. Pharmacol., 45:70.

17. Chang, T.M.S., Pont, A., Johnson, L.J., et al. Response to intermittent extracorporeal perfusion through shunts containing semipermeable microcapsules. Trans. Amer. Soc. Artif. Int. Organs, 15:163, 1968.

18. Chang, T.M.S. and Malave,N. The development and first clinical use of semipermeable microcapsules (artificial cells) as a compact artificial kidney. Trans. Amer. Soc. Artif. Int. Organs, 16:141, 1970.

19. Chang, T.M.S., Gonda, A., Dirks, J.H., and Malave, N. Clinical evaluation of chronic, internittent and short term hemoperfusion in patients with chronic renal failure using semipermeable microcapsules (artificial cells) formed from membrane-coated activated charcoal. Trans. Amer. Soc. Artif. Int. Organs, 17:246, 1971.

20. Chang, T.M.S., Gonda, A., Dirks, J.H., Coffey, J.F., and Lee-Burns,T. ACAC microcapsule artificial kidney for the long term and short term management of eleven patients with chronic renal failure. Trans. Amer. Soc. Artif. Int. Organs, 18:465, 1972.

21. Chang, T.M.S. Microcapsule artificial kidney: possible relationship between high clearance of medium molecular weight molecules and rapid alleviation of uremic symptoms. Proc. Eur. Dialysis Transplant Assoc., 9:568, 1972.

22. Chang T.M.S. and Migchelsen, M. Characterisation of Possible "Toxic" Metabolites in Uremia and Hepatic Coma based on the clearance spectrum for larger molecules by the ACAC microcapsule artificial kidney 19:314, 1973.

23. Chang, T.M.S., Coffey, J.F., Barre, P., Gonda, A., Dirks, J.H., Levy, M., and Lister, C. Microcapsule artificial kidney: treatment of patients with acute drug intoxication. C.M.A.J., 108:429, 1973.

24. Chang, T.M.S., Coffey, J.F., Lister, C., Taroy, E., and Stark, A., Methaqualone, Methyprylon, and Glutethemide clearance by the ACAC microcapsule artificial kidney in-vitre and in patients with acute intoxication. 19:87, 1973.

25.  Falb, R.D., Anapakos, P.G., Nack, H., and Kin, B.C. (1968):
     Feasibility of a microcapsule system for artificial kidney
     application. Annual Report, Artificial Kidney Program,
     National Institute of Health.

26.  Flinn, J.E., and Cherry, R.H.,Jr. (1970) Separation technology.
     Chem. Eng. Progr. Symp. Series, 65:90.

27.  Gardner, D.L. (1971): Possible uremic detoxification via oral
     ingested microcapsules. Trans. Amer. Soc. Artif. Intern.
     Organs (in press).

28.  Kitajima, M., Miyano, S., and Kondo, A. (1969): Studies on
     enzyme-containing microcapsules. J. Chem. Soc. Japan (Kogyo
     Kagaku Zasshi), 72:493.

29.  Kioshi, M., Fukuhara, N., and Kondo, T. (1968): Preparation
     of polyphthalamide microcapsules. Chem. Pharm. Bull., 17:804.

30.  Luzzi, L.A., (1970): Preparation and evaluation of the pro-
     longed release properties of nylon microcapsules, J. Pharm.
     Sci., 59:338.

31.  Sparks, R.E., Salemme, R.M., Meier, P.M., Litt, M.H., and
     Lindan, O. (1969): Removal of waster metabolites in uremia
     by microencapsulation reactants. Trans. Amer. Soc. Artif.
     Intern. Organs, 15:353.

32.  Sparks, R.E., Lindan, O., Mason, N.S., Litt, M.H., and Meier,
     P.M. (1971): Removal of uremic waste metabolites from the
     gastrointestinal tract by encapsulated carbon and oxidized
     starch. Trans. Amer. Soc. Artif. Intern. Organs (in press).

# MICROENCAPSULATION BY VAPOR DEPOSITION

William M. Jayne, Jr.

Union Carbide Corporation

Bound Brook, New Jersey

## SUMMARY

Encapsulation of particulate solids and of liquid droplets is commonly done for purposes of controlled release, environmental protection or rendering inert reactive, toxic, or hazardous materials. Coating of pharmaceuticals, pesticides, catalysts and discrete electronic elements are some specific examples of applications involving microencapsulation techniques. While most microencapsulation methods use liquid techniques, vapor-phase deposition of polymeric coatings using poly-p-xylylene is accomplished dry in vacuum environment. Encapsulation of substrates is accomplished by tumbling the particulate charge within an evacuated cylinder. Liquids are formed in droplets, frozen, and held at temperatures below their melting point during the subsequent coating operation. Deposition of poly-p-xylylene polymer from the reactive xylylene vapors uniformly coats and encapsulates the tumbling particles. Any desired thickness may be attained, from a few angstroms to over 1 mil if required for specific end-use. Examples will be discussed illustrating use and performance of encapsulated liquid and solid chemical materials.

## INTRODUCTION

Microencapsulation of liquids and solid particulates is conventionally done in liquid systems. Polymerization of the encapsulant barrier upon dispersed droplets or suspended solids takes place until reaction ceases due to buildup of a chemically impervious layer. Limitations to application of liquid techniques relate to needed mutual insolubility of the dispersed and carrier media, possible reactivity considerations and relative density of the two phases.

Encapsulation by means of vapor deposition using the poly-p-xylylene family of polymers is effected in a vacuum environment without a liquid carrier. They were first reported by Szwarc(1) in 1947 using xylene as the starting material. Later Gorham(2,3) showed that improved polymer quality and process control could be achieved by vacuum pyrolysis of di-p-xylylene. This family of polymers has been given the generic name of parylene.

## DISCUSSION

In contrast to other vapor-phase polymerization methods such as glow-discharge, electron beam and UV-initiation, formation of polymerizing species is conducted remotely from the deposition area. Pyrolytic cleavage of the dimer results in monomeric p-xylylene which is extremely reactive and polymerizes spontaneously upon contact with cool surfaces(4). Many chemical derivatives of di-p-xylylene have been synthesized, many of which can be converted to polymer in analogous fashion(2,5). Of particular interest for microencapsulation is poly(chloro-p-xylylene).

Physical properties of the parylenes make them attractive choices for use where their superior chemical resistance, low moisture permeability and high use temperature are of importance. The parylenes are insoluble in organic solvents at temperatures below 100°C and are unaffected by most acids and alkalis. Chlorinated hydrocarbons and strong oxidizers attack and dissolve the parylenes at elevated temperatures. Table I, following, gives some of the important physical property and permeability data on the parylenes.

### The Parylene Process

The starting material, di-p-xylylene,is placed in the vaporizer section of the apparatus as shown in Figures 1 and 2. Substrate, in this case in the form of particulate solid, is charged to the tumbler mounted on a rotatable fixture within the deposition chamber. Evacuation of the system to a pressure of less than 0.02 Torr is effected using a conventional mechanical vacuum pump preceded by a trap cooled by liquid nitrogen. The pyrolysis section is heated to a temperature of between 650 and 690°C prior to actual coating operation. Rotation of the partially filled tumbler is started as heat is applied to the vaporizer. Control of deposition rate of polymer on the cascading particulate charge is accomplished through control of vaporizer input power by means of system pressure measured at the exit of the pyrolysis zone by thermocouple type vacuum gauge probes. These probes are calibrated(6) for the particular parylene

## TABLE I

| Property | Parylene N | Parylene C |
|---|---|---|
| Structure | $\left[\!-CH_2-\!\bigcirc\!-CH_2-\!\right]_n$ | $\left[\!-CH_2-\!\underset{Cl}{\bigcirc}\!-CH_2-\!\right]_n$ |
| Tensile Strength, psi | 9,000 | 12,000 |
| Elongation to Break, % | 25 | 250 |
| Tensile Modulus, psi | 350,000 | 400,000 |
| Density, g/cc | 1.12 | 1.29 |
| Coefficient of Thermal Expansion in/in x $10^{-5}/^{\circ}C$ | 6.9 | 3.5 |
| Continuous Use Temperature, $^{\circ}C$ | | |
| in air | 100 | 120 |
| in vacuum | 220 | 225 |
| Gas Permeability cc-mil/100 $in^2$-24 hrs. | | |
| $N_2$ | 7.7 | 1.0 |
| $O_2$ | 39 | 7.2 |
| $CO_2$ | 214 | 7.7 |
| $Cl_2$ | 74 | 0.4 |
| Moisture Vapor Transmission g-mil/100 $in^2$-24 hrs. | 1.6 | 0.5 |

monomer in use and are maintained at $275^{\circ}C$ to retard polymer deposition within the gauge. Empirical relationships are used to determine dimer charge required for a given substrate surface area to achieve the desired thickness of encapsulant.

## Parylene Microencapsulation Applications

Microencapsulation using parylene polymers has been useful in three areas; inerting of reactive chemicals and controlled activity of catalysts, abrasion and atmospheric corrosion protection of electronic components and for placement of synthetic raindrops for missile reentry studies.

## APPARATUS FOR ENCAPSULATION OF PARTICULATE MATERIALS:

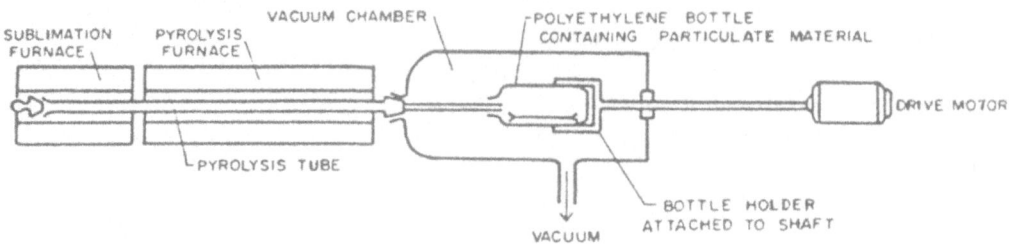

FIGURE 1

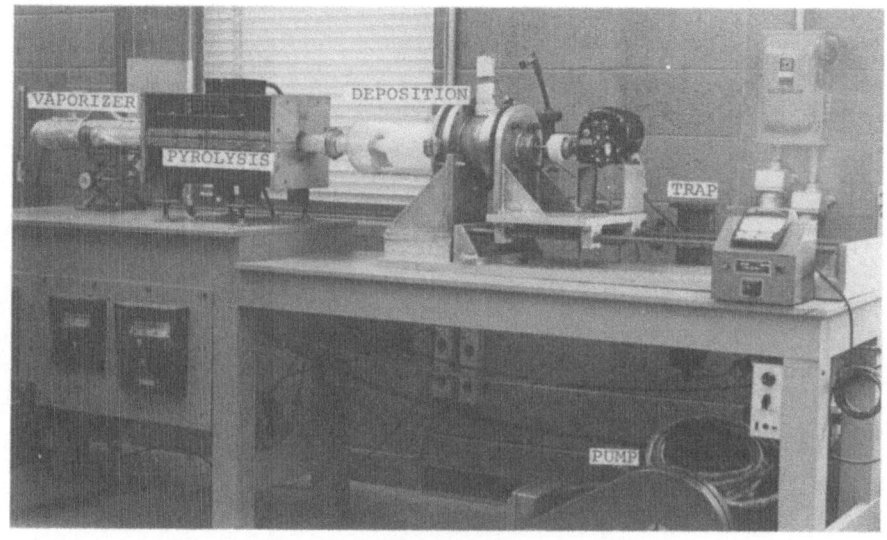

FIGURE 2

Parylene Encapsulation Equipment

## Reactive Chemical Encapsulation

While many types of reactive chemical materials have been encapsulated using the parylenes, the encapsulation of lithium metal is discussed here as a typical case(7). Parylene C was chosen as the encapsulating polymer because of its low moisture vapor permeability. Three different thicknesses of polymer were applied to the lithium metal shot used. Degree of protection was established by exposing the coated lithium to atmospheres controlled at three different relative humidities using pure water, saturated NaCl and saturated MgCl$_2 \cdot$6H$_2$0. Steady-state hydrogen evolution measured using a U-tube manometer gave indication of protection provided by the encapsulant polymer. As shown in Table II, the coating does indeed provide substantial reduction in rate of reaction in comparison to bare lithium from 10 fold for the 0.5 micron coating to nearly 400 fold for 7 micron barriers.

TABLE II

| Coating Thickness Microns | Relative Humidity (RH) | Steady-State Hydrogen Evolution per Unit Area (mm/hr/cm$^2$) |
|---|---|---|
| 0 | 100 | 2.078 |
| 0 | 76 | 0.945 |
| 0.5 | 100 | 0.197 |
| 0.5 | 76 | 0.165 |
| 0.5 | 33 | 0.102 |
| 2.3 | 100 | 0.028 |
| 2.3 | 76 | 0.022 |
| 2.3 | 33 | 0.0067 |
| 7.0 | 100 | 0.0056 |
| 7.0 | 76 | 0.0045 |
| 7.0 | 33 | 0.0025 |

Many other reactive materials have been encapsulated using the parylene process as shown in Table III. Liquids such as aromatic solvents and water or aqueous solutions can also be successfully encapsulated. Figure 3 shown microcapsules of xylene initially prepared using coacervation techniques. A small paper clip is included for size comparison. An overcoating of 0.5 mils of parylene C applied by tumbling served to decrease loss of the volatile xylenes by more than 10 fold. Seven years after coating the microcapsules retain 90% of their original contents. Storage conditions were 25$^o$C in a covered but not sealed glass container. Handling of normally liquid materials in the parylene process generally requires freezing in the desired particulate shape prior to coating.

TABLE III

Solid Materials Encapsulated with the Parylenes

| | |
|---|---|
| Salts | NaCl |
| | $CaCl_2$ |
| Bases | NaOH |
| | KOH |
| Reducing Agents | $LiAlH_4$ |
| Oxidizing Agents | $NH_4ClO_4$ |
| | $KMnO_4$ |
| Metals | Zn |
| | Na |
| | K |
| | Li |

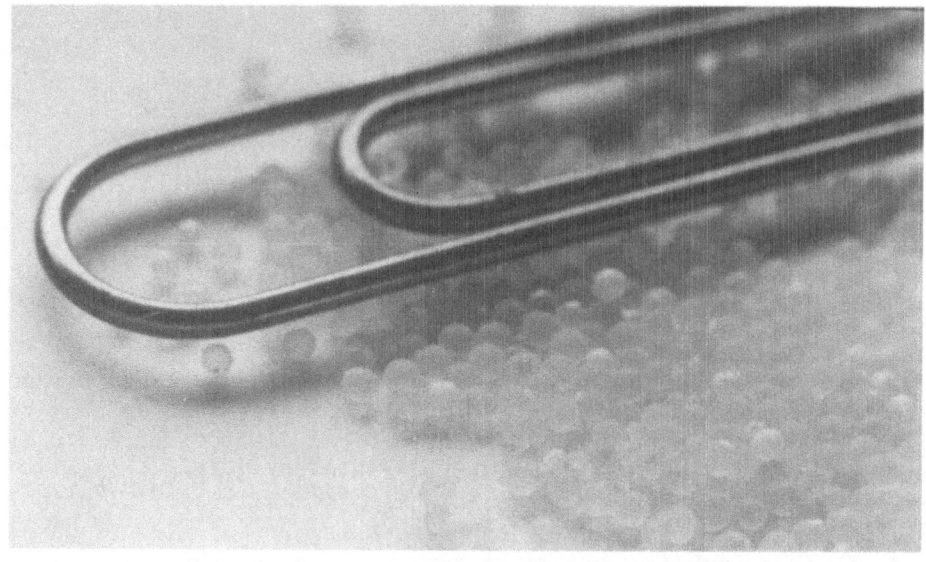

FIGURE 3

Encapsulated Xylene Droplets

The tumbler assembly must, in these cases, be cooled to slightly below the normal liquid freezing point to minimize offgassing or boiling so that the polymer shell can form and contain the substrate. Control of encapsulant shell thickness has been shown to provide controlled release of reactive or volatile materials as desired for particular end-uses.

### Corrosion Protection-Electronics

Encapsulation of many types of miniature electronic components and assemblies is being done using parylene systems. Encapsulation of particulates as opposed to fixtured circuit boards is typified by the coating of ferrite computer memory cores as shown in Figure 4(8).

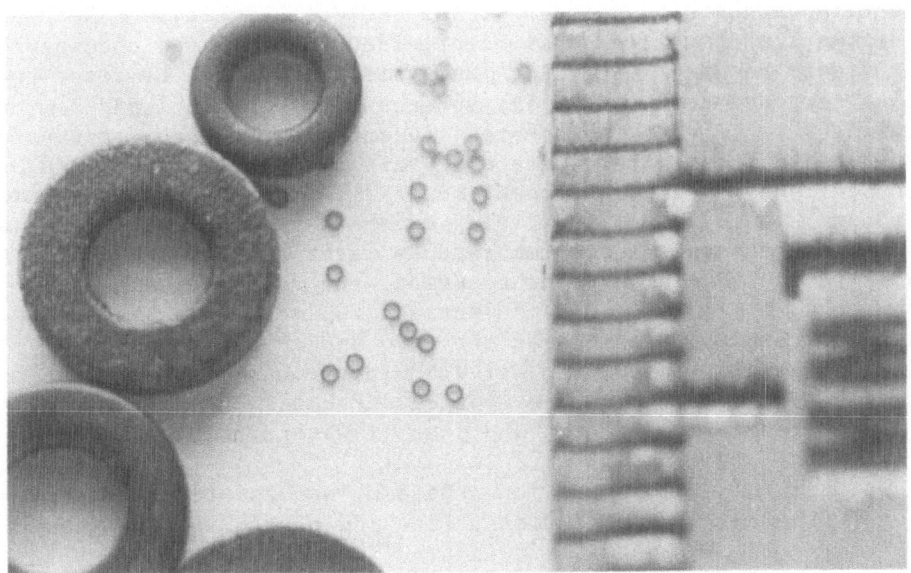

FIGURE 4

Encapsulated Ferrite Toroids

These devices in the shape of doughnuts from 1 mm to 10 mm in outside diameter have been encapsulated with from 0.1 to 1 mil of parylenes N and C. The main purpose of the encapsulant was to prevent cut-through of the insulation on wires subsequently passed through the toroids during memory fabrication. Parylene's outstanding abrasion resistance has been effective in preventing damage to insulating enamels on such devices, such that shorts are eliminated. Normal coating thicknesses of about 0.5 mil have proven adequate in this application.

Corrosion effects due to atmospheric attack of electronic components in hostile environments are effectively prevented by parylene encapsulation. While much of this work is better represented as macro rather than microencapsulation, tumble coating of miniature components has been done.

### Rain and Dust Screens for Missile Reentry Studies

Recent application of microencapsulation using the parylene system has been in the construction of synthetic rain and dust environments for missile reentry studies. Testing of spacecraft and missile ablative materials by Naval Ordnance Laboratory in Silver Spring, Maryland requires exposure of missile materials to atmospheres containing raindrops, ice and dust particles. Reproducible arrays of particles must be provided to allow valid comparisons of candidate reentry materials. Rain arrays are made by first tumble coating screened urea $(CO(NH_2)_2)$ spheres with between 1 and 3 microns of parylene C. The coated spheres are attached in spaced arrays on clean glass plates. The entire array and plate are coated with 0.2 microns of parylene and the resulting film with attached urea beads lifted and mounted on a target ring as shown in Figure 5. Numbers of such mounted screens are immersed in water as they are needed for missile tests. During a 48 hour period, the urea is leached out through the thin polymer encapsulant and replaced with water. The patterned "raindrop" screens as they now appear are mounted as shown in Figure 6, in 100% relative humidity chambers within the test range. Chamber doors are kept closed until just prior to test firing to prevent evaporation and loss of water from the screens.

Ice screens are made in much the same way as are the rain screens. The only exception being freezing of the screens just prior to testing.

Dust arrays are made from glass beads, so require no tumble coating prior to patterning and mounting on target rings, nor any special further treatment prior to firing tests.

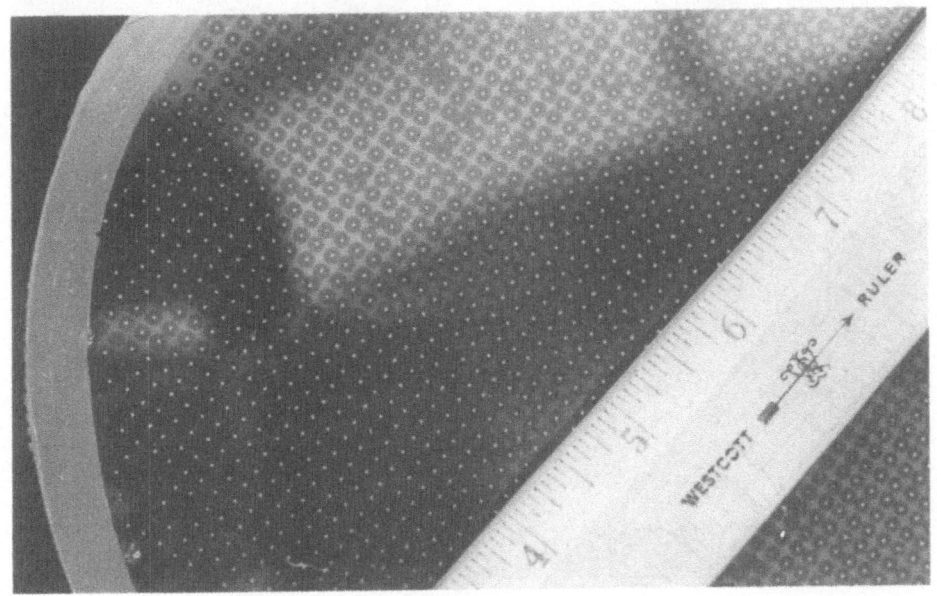

FIGURE 5

8 Inch Synthetic Rain Screen
Showing Patterned, Encapsulated Urea Beads

In the above application, parylene serves two functions: (1) permits mounting of precisely sized water or particulate water in a fixed, reproducible pattern and (2) provides a very low-mass means of supporting the particles. Particle sizes of from 0.2 mm to 1.2 mm have been used, yielding particle-to-support mass ratios of between about 200 and 1000:1.

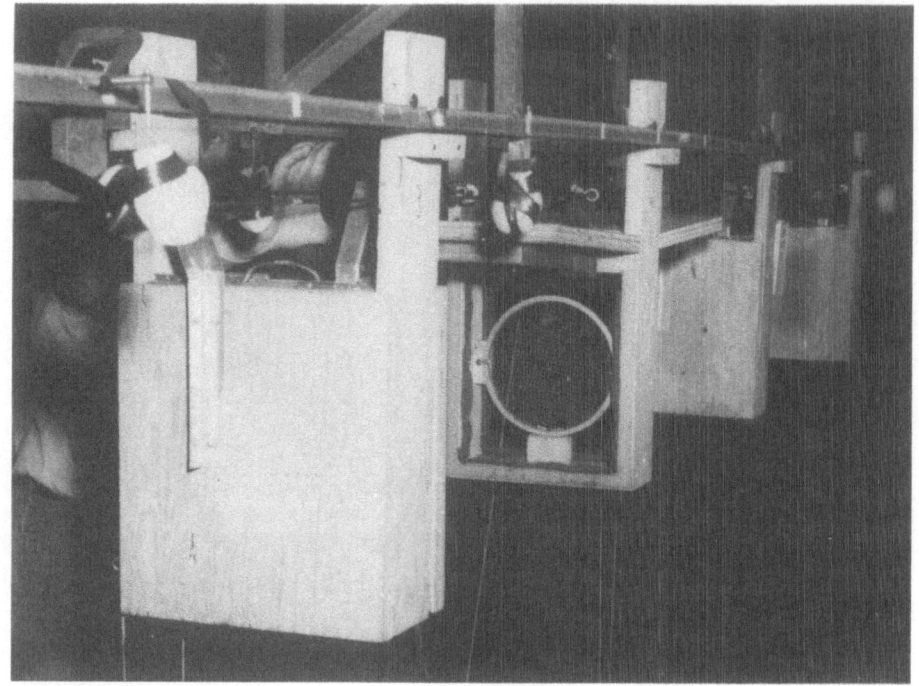

FIGURE 6

Naval Ordnance Laboratory Firing Range Showing
Rain Screen in Position in Open Humidity Chamber

CONCLUSION

Microencapsulation using vacuum deposition of parylene polymers
can provide unique products for applications requiring controlled
release, environmental protection and specific mechanical or chemical properties.  Coatings on solid particulates may be applied in
thicknesses from a few angstroms to several mils to provide desired
barrier permeability or mechanical properties.

REFERENCES

(1) M. Szwarc, Discussion Faraday Soc. 2, 46 (1947).
(2) W. F. Gorham, J. Poly. Sci. A-1, 4, 3027 (1966).
(3) W. F. Gorham, U. S. 3,342,754.

(4) S. W. Chow, W. E. Loeb and C. E. White, J. Appl.
    Polym. Sci., 13, 2325 (1969).

(5) W. F. Gorham, U. S. 3,288,728.

(6) M. A. Spivack, D. B. Anderson, L. L. Carpenter,
    J. Vac. Sci. and Technology 6, 5, 859 (1969).

(7) M. A. Spivack, Corrosion, 26, 9, 371 (1970).

(8) J. H. Magee and R. D. Fisher, IEEE Trans. on
    Magnetics Mag.-6, 1, 34 (1970).

# MICROENCAPSULATION OF ACTIVATED CHARCOAL

# AND ITS BIOCHEMICAL APPLICATIONS

Masataka Morishita, Mitsuri Fukushima and Yoshihito Inaba

Research Laboratories, Toyo Jozo Co. Ltd.

Mifuku, Ohito-cho, Shizuoka-ken, 410-23, Japan

## Introduction

Since Emmett[1] reported the molecular sieving effect of carbonated saran, various types of molecular sieving carbons have been prepared and used in the chemical industry. Recently, Chang et.al.[2]-[5] reported activated charcoal microcapsules having semipermeable membranes such as collodion or nylon and their application in an artificial kidney. The authors report the preparation, properties, molecular sieving characteristics, and some biochemical applications of polymer-encapsulated, activated charcoal microcapsules which have been developed in their laboratories.

## Materials and Methods

### Preparation of activated charcoal microcapsules

The following three methods of microencapsulation were used to prepare activated charcoal microcapsules. Activated coconut charcoal powder of 150-500 mesh (Takeda Chemical Industries Co. Ltd.) was used in all cases.

### 1) Complex emulsion method (Evaporation of the solvent in water)

Activated charcoal powder was dispersed uniformly in a polymer solution of a water-immiscible volatile solvent such as methylene-chloride or chloroform. This dispersion was poured into an aqueous vehicle containing an anionic surface active agent to form small uniform droplets under stirring. In this case gelatin is not suitable, because in gelatin, activated charcoal coagulates.

Under stirring, uniform droplets are formed; the size of these
droplets determine the size of microcapsules.  After continuous
stirring for 8-10 hours at room temperature and if necessary
warming up in a water bath, the solvent evaporates and a rigid
polymer film forms around the charcoal.  After separation from
the aqueous solution, the capsules are washed repeatedly in water
and dried in a ventilated oven at 50°C.  The microcapsules thus
obtained are spherical grains having diameters of 0.3-1.5mm.

FIGURE 1

Microencapsulation process in the complex emulsion method

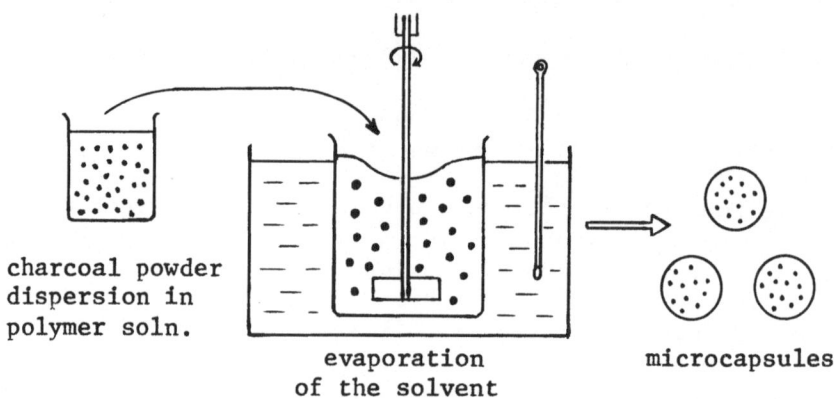

charcoal powder          evaporation          microcapsules
dispersion in            of the solvent
polymer soln.

### 2) Droplet formation method (Orifice method)

In this method, dimethylformamide or dimethylsulfoxide was
used as the polymer solvent.  Charcoal powder was added to the
polymer solution (10% w/v) and this uniform dispersion added drop-
wise to an aqueous coagulating bath by means of an atomizer cup.
The size of the microcapsules could be controlled by the running
speed of the atomizer cup and by the viscosity of the polymer
solution.  As soon as the droplets contacted water, gel formation
occurred at the interface.  After standing overnight in water, the
solvent was replaced by water.  Capsules obtained in this way
could not be dried; it was necessary to store them in a wet
condition.  Microcapsules thus obtained have diameters of
1.0-5.0mm.

### 3) Pearl Polymerization method (Emulsion polymerization in non-polar solvent)

According to the published methods, polysaccharide such as
dextran or dextrin was polymerized to form microcapsules containing
activated charcoal powder.  Charcoal powder was dispersed in an
alkaline dextran solution, then poured into liquid paraffin and

FIGURE 2
Microencapsulation process in the droplet formation method

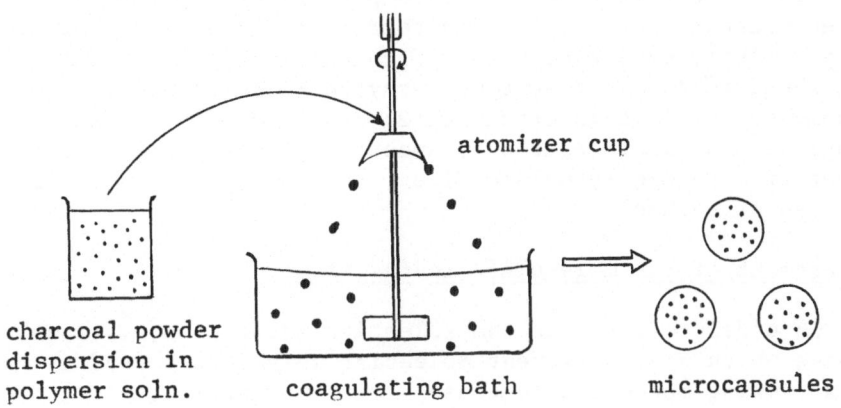

stirred to make a water in oil emulsion.  Epichlorohydrin, a crosslinking agent, was added to this emulsion and the reaction mixture
was maintained at 50°C under agitation.  After completion of the
reaction, the produced microcapsules were washed with n-hexane and
acetone and then with water until neutrality.

FIGURE 3
Microencapsulation process in the pearl polymerization method

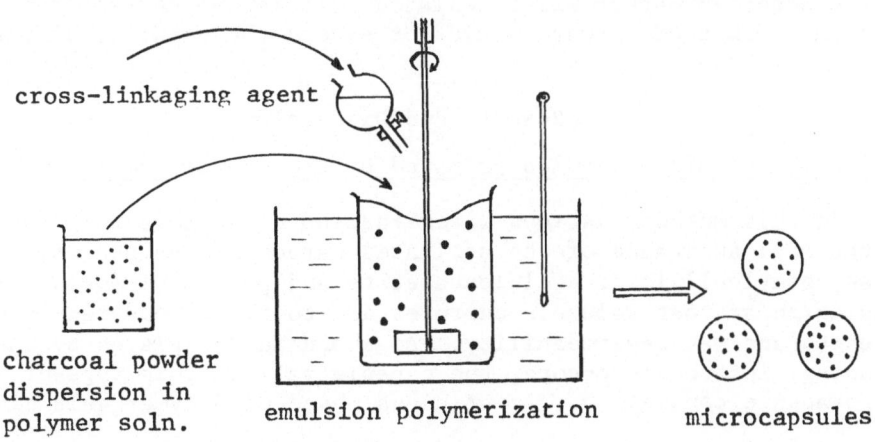

## Determination of the adsorption capacity

The adsorption capacity was measured by using methylene-blue and caramel as test substances, comparing the capsules with non-coated charcoal powder and some commercial bead type charcoals. Various microcapsules,each sample containing 1g of charcoal powder, were added to 100ml of aqueous methylene-blue solution (0.01% w/v, OD595m$\mu$ =5.50). At intervals of 24 and 48 hours, non-adsorbed methylene-blue was measured by spectrophotometry to calculate an amount of adsorbed methylene-blue. The same process was used in the case of caramel.

## Measurement of the molecular sieving effect

In order to estimate the selective adsorption, various substances which have different molecular weight were used as markers, The following markers were chosen for their affinity to activated charcoal and their ease of detection.

Methylene-blue (MW=374), Tuberactinomycin (MW=798), Polymixin B (MW-1,280), Insulin (MW-5,700), Lysozyme (MW=14,000), $\alpha$-chymo-trypsin (MW=24,500). Semi-alkaline proteinase (MW=30,000), Pepsin (MW=35,000), Ovo-albumin (MW=45,000), Serum albumin (MW-67,000), $\gamma$ -Globulin (MW-156,000).

Of these markers, Methylene-blue was detected by measuring the optical density at 595m$\mu$ , Polymixin B by measuring antibiotic potency, and others by measuring optical density at 280m$\mu$. Ten ml of each marker solution (100mg-12.5mg/10ml of water) was charged on the column ($\emptyset$=1cm) which had been packed with microencapsulated activated charcoal containing 1g of non-coated activated charcoal at the flow rate of 0.5ml/min, and the eluate was fractionated in 5ml fractions. The column was washed out with water until the marker was no longer detectable in the eluate. The amount of marker in each fraction was measured, summed, and then the amount of the adsorbed marker was calculated. It is, of course, necessary that the amount of marker should not exceed the capacity of the column.

## Results and Discussion

## Evaluation of microcapsules prepared by the complex emulsion method

In this method, various water insoluble polymers could be used as the wall substance of the activated carbon microcapsules. Among these, ethylcellulose, celluloseacetate and polyvinyl-formal were considered as most valuable capsules due to their good mechanical strength and water-permeability. As shown in the plates by the scanning electronmicroscope, the capsule wall in this type of microcapsule consists of a continuous phase of polymer gels having

a microporous structure with the carbon powder existing at inner-
side of the polymer-gel.  The pore structure is considered to be
made by the evaporation of the solvent during the preparation of
the microcapsules.

Plate 1
Electron microscope photograph
of Celluloseacetate capsule

Plate 2
Electronmicroscope photograph
of Polyvinylformal capsule

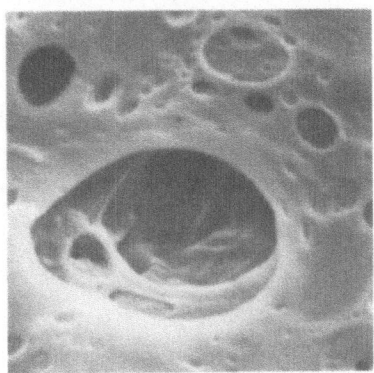        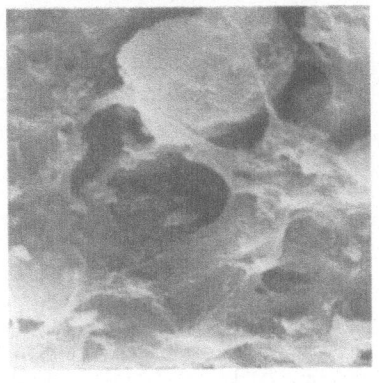

8,000 x magnification            2,400 x magnification

By the reason of such a structure, microcapsules prepared by
this method have a high adsorption capacity compared with some
commercial beads of charcoal.  The adsorption capacity measured by
methylene-blue method is shown in Table 1.

TABLE 1

Adsorption capacity of microcapsules prepared
by complex emulsion method

| Sample | 24 hours | | 48 hours | |
|---|---|---|---|---|
| | $OD_{595}$ | Adsorp.(%) | $OD_{595}$ | Adsorp.(%) |
| None | 5.500 | 0 | 5.500 | 0 |
| Charcoal powder | 0 | 100 | 0 | 100 |
| Ethylecellulose capsule | 0.542 | 90 | 0.341 | 94 |
| Celluloseacetate capsule | 0.320 | 94 | 0.057 | 99 |
| Polyvinylformal capsule | 0.648 | 88 | 0.078 | 99 |
| Commercial beads A | 1.900 | 65 | 1.650 | 70 |
| Commercial beads B | 1.850 | 66 | 1.030 | 81 |
| Commercial beads C | 2.950 | 46 | 0.984 | 82 |

0.01% methylene-blue solution was used as the marker.  Details are
described in the test.

The selective adsorption of the marker was tested on these microencapsulated charcoals using columns packed with them. The results are summarized in Figure 4 showing the clear molecular sieving effect of these preparations. About 30,000 in molecular weight is a boundary line of molecular sieving. If each micropore could take part in molecular sieving, the size of the pores would be about 25A based on the calculation of molecular size of semi-alkaline proteinase[6].

FIGURE 4

Molecular sieving effect of microcapsules
by the complex emulsion method

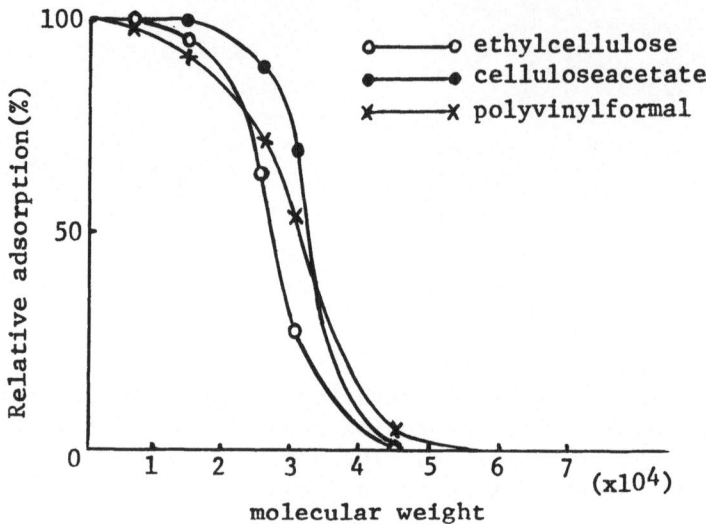

FIGURE 5

Structure of the microcapsule
prepared by droplet formation

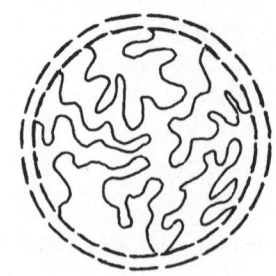

Evaluation of microcapsules prepared by the droplet formation method

Among the many polymers tested by this method, cellulose-acetate, polyacrylonitrile and vinylchloride-vinylacetate copolymer prove to have the most promise. The capsules prepared from these polymers had a smooth surface showing a microporous membrane structure contiguous to an inner polymer-gel loaded with water and of a sponge-like structure as shown in Figure 5.

TABLE 2
Adsorption capacity of microcapsules prepared
by droplet formation method

| Samples | 24 hours | | 48 hours | |
|---|---|---|---|---|
| | $OD_{595}m\mu$ | Adsorp.(%) | $OD_{595}m\mu$ | Adsorp.(%) |
| None | 5.000 | 0 | 5.000 | 0 |
| Charcoal powder | 0 | 100 | 0 | 100 |
| Celluloseacetate | 0.550 | 89 | 0.096 | 98 |
| " +detergent | 0.472 | 91 | 0.129 | 97 |
| Polyacrylonitrile | 0.635 | 87 | 0.153 | 97 |
| Vinyl Cl-vinyl Ac copolymer | 1.510 | 70 | 0.193 | 96 |
| Commertial beads A | 2.210 | 56 | 0.480 | 90 |
| " B | 2.950 | 41 | 0.984 | 80 |
| " C | 3.550 | 29 | 1.065 | 79 |

0.01% methylene-blue solution was used as the marker. Details are described in method.

TABLE 3
Adsorption capacity of microcapsule prepared
by droplet formation method

| Samples | 24 hours | | 48 hours | |
|---|---|---|---|---|
| | $OD_{420}m\mu$ | Adsorp.(%) | $OD_{420}m\mu$ | Adsorp.(%) |
| None | 4.320 | 0 | 4.320 | 0 |
| Charcoal powder | 1.570 | 100 | 1.390 | 100 |
| Celluloseacetate | 1.675 | 96 | 1.400 | 100 |
| +detergent | 1.655 | 97 | 1.460 | 98 |
| Polyacrylonitrile | 1.980 | 85 | 1.610 | 93 |
| Vinyl Cl-vinyl Ac copolymer | 2.170 | 78 | 2.030 | 78 |
| Commercial beads A | 2.650 | 61 | 2.500 | 62 |
| " B | 2.260 | 75 | 1.955 | 81 |
| " C | 3.700 | 23 | 3.650 | 23 |

Caramel solution ($OD_{420}m\mu$=4.320) was used as the marker. Details are described in method.

The advantage of this type of microcapsule is that its
molecular sieving effect depends only on the outer microporous
structure, and the molecules which pass through the membrane are
considered to difuse freely into the inner sponge-like gels and
reach the dispersed charcoal particles.  The capacity to adsorb
methylene-blue is much the same as that of capsules prepared by the
complex emulsion method, however, the adsorption of caramel is
superior than with other types of capsules by reason of their
higher permeability of the capsule wall (Tables 2 and 3).

The molecular sieving effect of these capsules is shown in
Figure 6.  It is quite remarkable that the range of the molecular
cutting-off could be moved about 10,000 lower by adding some
detergent to the polymer solution on its microencapsulation.

FIGURE 6

<u>Molecular sieving effect of the microcapsules prepared</u>
<u>by droplet formation method</u>

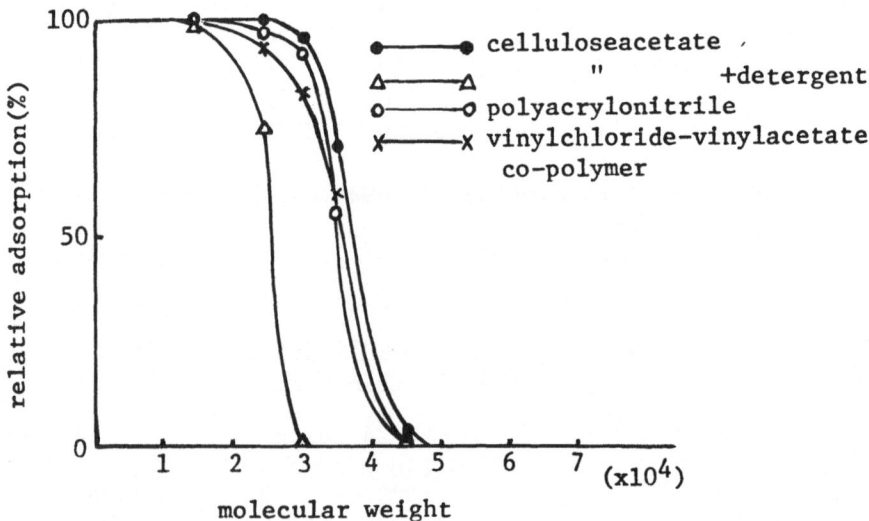

<u>Evaluation of microcapsules prepared by the pearl polymerization</u>
<u>method</u>

In this method, the wall material of the activated charcoal
microcapsules was selected from the polysaccharide group
represented by compounds such as dextran or dextrin.  The capsules
thus obtained were quite resistant to mechanical stress, but the
content of activated charcoal was less than with capsules prepared
by the other methods.

The excellent adsorption capacity of methylene-blue and the
sharpest molecular cut off characteristic were achieved by this
type of microcapsules as demonstrated in Table 4 and Figure 7.
The polymerization degree of dextran had no relation to the molecular sieving boundary line.

TABLE 4

Adsorption capacity of microcapsules prepared
by pearl polymerization method

| Samples | 24 hours | | 48 hours | |
|---|---|---|---|---|
| | OD595mμ | Adsorp.(%) | OD595mμ | Adsorp.(%) |
| None | 5.500 | 0 | 5.500 | 0 |
| Charcoal powder | 0 | 100 | 0 | 100 |
| Dextran(70,000) capsule | 0.021 | 99.6 | 0.005 | 99.9 |
| (40,000) capsule | 0.059 | 99.0 | 0.024 | 99.6 |
| (10,000) capsule | 0.106 | 98.1 | 0.029 | 99.5 |
| Dextrin capsule | 0.088 | 98.4 | 0.022 | 99.6 |
| Commercial beads A | 1.900 | 65.5 | 1.650 | 70.0 |
| " B | 1.850 | 66.4 | 1.030 | 81.3 |
| " C | 2.950 | 46.4 | 0.984 | 82.1 |
| " D | 3.500 | 35.5 | 1.065 | 80.6 |

0.01% methylene-blue solution was used as the marker.  Details are
described in method.

FIGURE 7

Molecular sieving effect of the microcapsules prepared
by pearl polymerization method

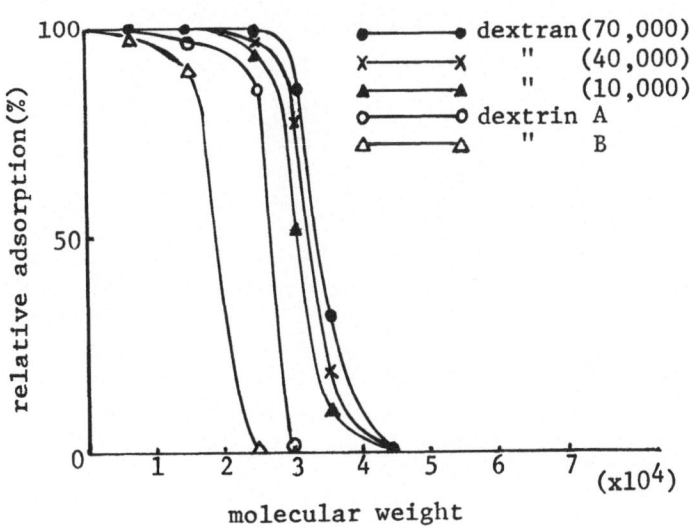

## Characteristics of activated charcoal microcapsules

The most outstanding feature of the activated charcoal microcapsules described above is their clearly specific molecular
sieving effect.  In contrast with other molecular sieving polymers
such as Sephadex and Bio-gel, these microcapsules have a large
adsorption capacity, larger than any other commercial beads of
carbon.

This unique tool can be furnished, by reason of the combination of molecular sieving effect of polymers with the strong
adsorption activity of charcoal.  Thereby, it has become possible
to efficiently separate a variety of organic substances.

## Biochemical applications of activated charcoal microcapsules

The following applications of the microcapsules prepared by
the abovementioned methods were studied.

1)  Purification of kanamycin from Broth filtrate
One hundred sixty ml of broth filtrate containing 80mg
(potency) kanamycin were charged on a column (1cm x 16cm) which had
been filled with 3.3g of ethylcellulose microcapsules (ethylcellulose 40%, activated charcoal powder 60%) prepared by the complex
emulsion method.  All the kanamycin in the broth filtrate was
adsorbed on the microcapsules but other components of the medium
such as glucose, polypepton, and melanoid pigment were not adsorbed
and passed through the column.  After repeated washing with distilled water, kanamycin was eluted with 0.01 N-HCl-methanol (1:1).
The eluate was colorless and the recovery of kanamycin was 72.8mg
(p).  (Yield=91%)  The amount of kanamycin was measured by
bioassay.

### FIGURE 8
Purification of kanamycin from Broth filtrate

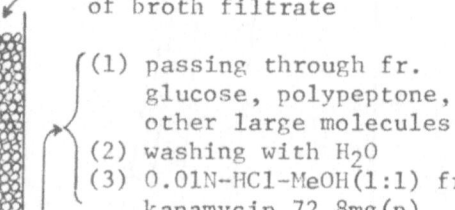

M.C. prepared
by complex
emulsion method
(ethyl cellulose
40%, A.C. powder
60%) 3.3g

— 80mg(p) kanamycin in 160ml
   of broth filtrate

(1) passing through fr.
    glucose, polypeptone,
    other large molecules
(2) washing with $H_2O$
(3) 0.01N-HCl-MeOH(1:1) fr.
    kanamycin 72.8mg(p)

2)   Purification of tuberactinomycin from broth filtrate.

In the same procedure 75.3mg of tuberactinomycin were separated from 50ml of broth filtrate (2.26mg (p)/ml) on a column filled with 2.5g of polyvinylformal microcapsules (polyvinylformal) 20% activated charcoal powder 80%) prepared by the complex emulsion method.  (Yield=67%)

3)   Decolorization of protease solution

Fermentation broth filtrate containing alkaline protease (MW=30,000) was passed through a column of cellulose acetate-detergent capsules made by the droplet formation method.  The optical density at 420mµ of the solution decreased from 0.680 to 0.068 on passage through the volumn, but 67% of proteolytic activity was recovered.

4)   Decolorization of Japanese sake

Sake has a color of pale yellow, and powdered charcoal is used for decolorization now, but it is not convenient.  By using the column of charcoal microcapsules prepared by the droplet formation method, the process can be made continuous.  After checking the clarity, acid content, and taste of the eluate, we find that we have pretty good results.  Polyacrylonitrile is the most useful material for the capsule wall in this application.

5)   Extraction of caramel pigment from alcohol fermentation waste.

Molasses is used in alcohol fermentation, and we have tried to recover caramel pigment from the waste, by using a column of poly-acrylonitrile capsules.  After passing through an ion exchange column, the waste was charged on the microcapsule column at pH 4.0 and washed out with water.  The caramel pigment was then eluted with 0.5N-ammonia water.  Upon concentration of this solution, very good caramel was obtained.

6)   Purification of lysozyme from egg white.

Twenty five ml of fresh egg white was diluted with distilled water to 300ml, and homogenized in a Waring blender.  After the foam was removed by centrifuge, 20ml of the solution was charged on the column, (1cm x 18cm) which was filled with 3g of dextrin microcapsules (content of activated charcoal powder was about 22%) and then eluted with distilled water and 0.1N-HCl.  The eluate was fractionated in 10ml portions.  The elution diagram is shown in Figure 9.

In the early stage of elution, ovo-albumin, con-albumin, ovo-globulin, ovo-mucoid and ovo-mutin which were contained in the egg white were passed through the column and only lysozyme was retained by the charcoal.  In the later stage, lysozyme was eluted out completely with 0.1N-HCl.  In this purification, the activity yield of lysozyme was determined by the lysis of M. lysodeikticus.

FIGURE 9
Elution diagram of column chromatography of egg white

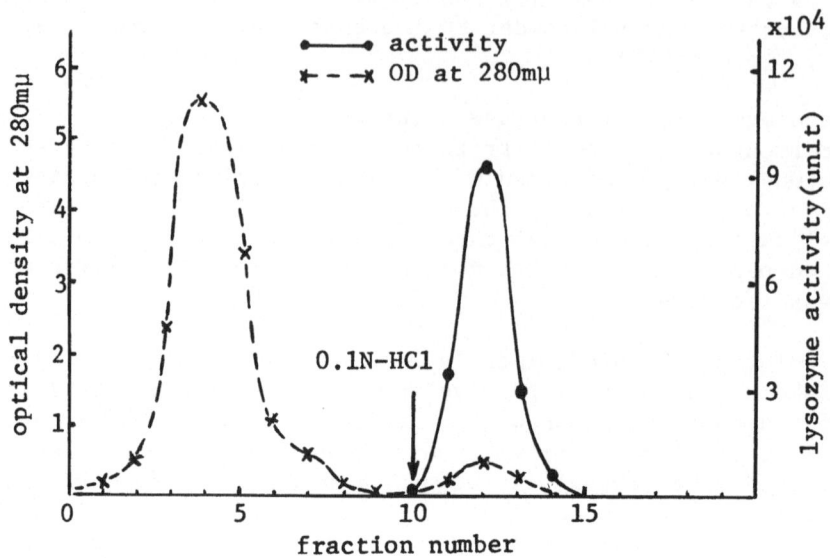

Aknowledgement

The authors wish to express their sincere thanks to Dr. Asashi Kondo, Fuji Photofilm Co. Ltd., for his kind discussion and encouragement throughout the present study.

References

1) Emmett, P.H. ; Chem. Rev., 43 69 (1948)
2) Chang, T.M.S. ; Science, 146 524 (1964)
3) Chang, T.M.S. ; Trans. Amer. Soc. Artif. Intern. Organs, 12 13 (1964)
4) Chang, T.M.S., Macintosh, F.C., and Mason, S.G. ; Can. J. Physiol. Pharmacol., 44 115 (1966)
5) Chang, T.M.S., Pont, A., Johnson, L.J., and Malvave, N. Trans. Amer. Soc. Artif. Intern. Organs, 14 163 (1968)
6) Sugiura and Ito ; Yakugaku Zasshi, 88 1591 (1968)

# MICROENCAPSULATION PROCESSES IN MODERN BUSINESS FORMS

George Baxter

Moore Business Forms, Inc.
Research Division
1001 Buffalo Avenue
Niagara Falls, New York    14302

The application of microencapsulation technology to pressure sensitive copying systems in modern manifold business forms has grown dramatically in the past few years.  It appears that the higher cost and higher waste during forms manufacture with such systems have become less significant factors in curtailing their use than they were formerly.  The improved quality and cleanliness of the copy obtained with microcapsule systems as compared with the older hot melt wax (carbon paper) systems is only a partial explanation for their wider use.  Short supply of raw materials, preservation of the ecology and waste disposal are now serious considerations limiting the use of the older pressure transfer copying systems.  The technical and economic feasibility of recycling carbonless copying papers after use has been demonstrated and this is an additional attractive feature of such systems.

## Requirements of Microcapsules for Use in Carbonless Copying

The encapsulation processes described here were developed specifically for business forms applications which limit the microcapsules' size to the 1-10 microns range (Figure 1).  There is no reason why these processes could not be modified or adapted to produce a larger sized capsule, however. In all of the processes the first step is to produce a stable emulsion of the material to be encapsulated in a continuous phase comprising the film former or a component of the film former material capable of forming the shell of the capsules.  It is also desirable to have the microcapsules in the form of a dry, free-flowing powder for ease and versatility of application to paper or other substrates.  This can generally be achieved with these processes by spray-drying or simple filtration and drying in some cases.

The essential characteristic of the film-former, of course, is
that it be insoluble in the material to be encapsulated. Also, the
capsule wall should be non-porous, to contain and protect the
active capsule contents, and abrasion resistant, to prevent premature rupture due to incidental scuffing. A capsule wall having
the physical characteristics of an egg shell would be a fairly
ideal structure. The capsule wall should also protect the contents
from environmental factors such as humidity and temperature variations, and the possible presence of other reactive or potentially
harmful materials. All of the processes to be discussed encapsulate
a liquid core since this is preferred in copying systems because of
its superior pressure transfer characteristics in comparison with
solid or semi-solid core materials.

## Microencapsulation by Spray-Drying

In this method, a stable emulsion is produced in which the
continuous phase contains a film-forming material capable of forming the capsule shell and which is insoluble in the marking fluid.
The discontinuous or dispersed phase of the emulsion constitutes

Microcapsule Size Range 1-10 microns

Non-Porous Thin Shell

Brittle Shell, Rupturable Under Pressure

Abrasion Resistant Shell

Shell Inert To Encapsulated Materials

Shell Resistant To Environmental Changes

Biodegradable Shell

Figure 1. Microcapsule requirements for carbonless copying.

the marking fluid, and comprises pigment, colored dye or colorless dye intermediate suspended or dissolved in a non-volatile liquid. The emulsion is then spray-dried, or the film-forming material is first condensed around the emulsified droplets by curing or other means, and then filtered and dried, or spray-dried. The resulting product is a dry, free-flowing powder. (Several modifications of this process are shown schematically in Figures 2, 4 and 5)

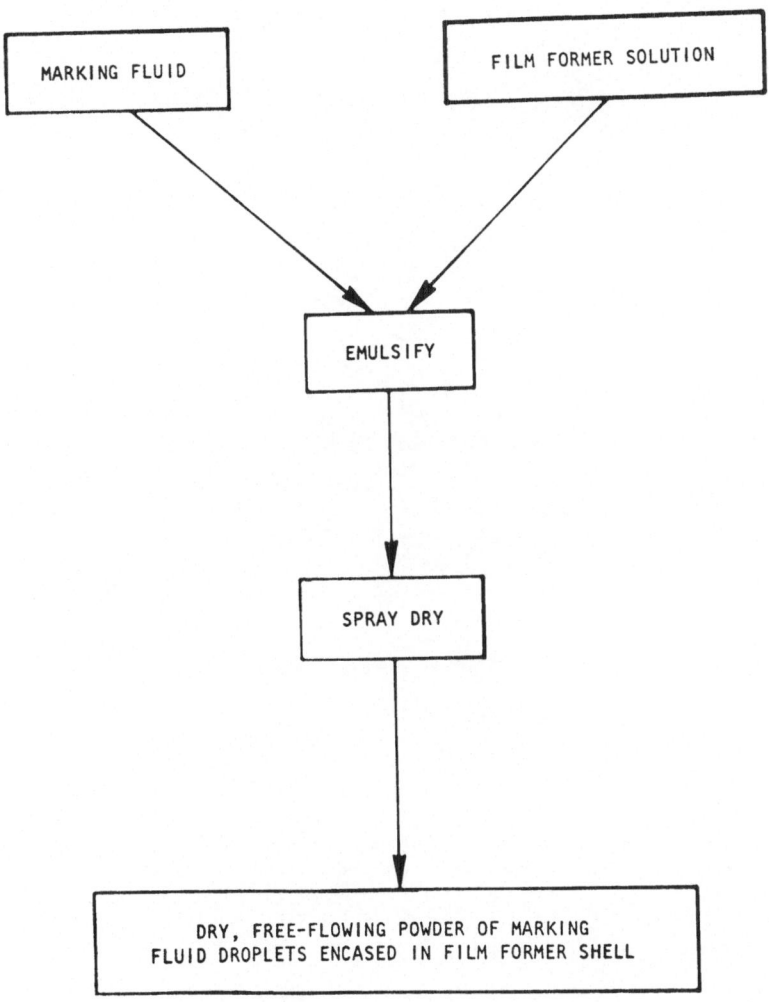

Figure 2. Microcapsule formation by spray-drying emulsion with dissolved film-former as continuous phase.

In the first process (Figure 2) microcapsules are produced by
spray-drying an emulsion with dissolved film-former as the continuous phase.  Some film-formers which are useful in the process
are casein, zein, carboxymethyl cellulose, methyl cellulose,
hydroxyethyl cellulose, cellulose acetate, petroleum hydrocarbon
resins and other synthetic resins.  Inorganic film formers such as
sodium silicate have been employed also, although such film-formers
are less desirable because of the difficulty of maintaining a
stable emulsion.  Figure 3 is a photomicrograph of microcapsules
obtained by spray-drying an emulsion of mineral oil in an aqueous
zein solution.

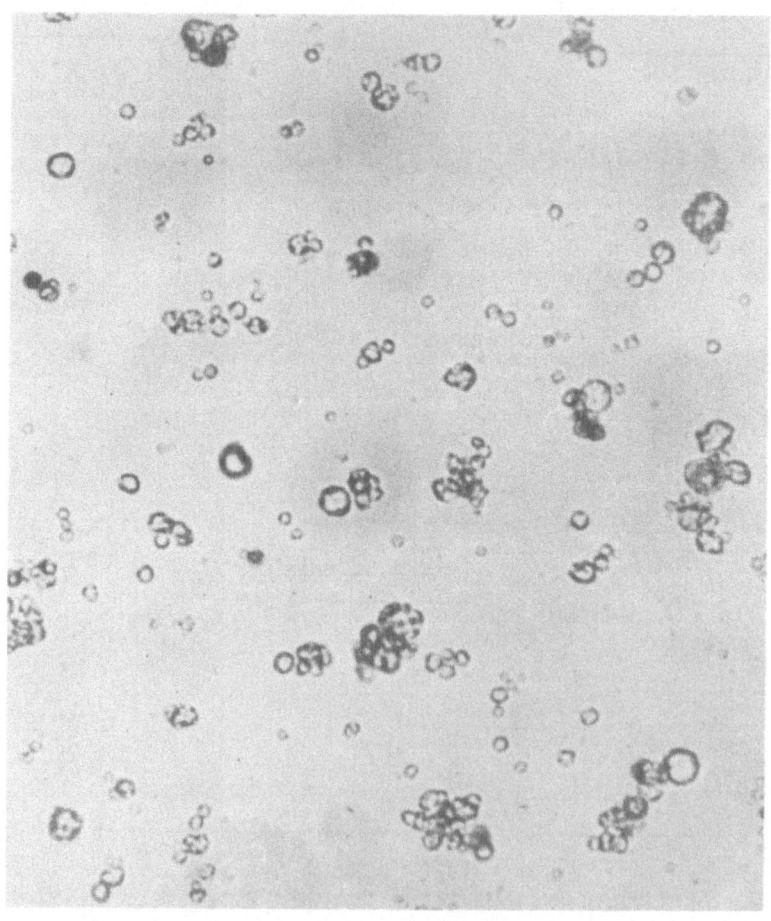

Figure 3.  Photomicrograph of zein/mineral oil microcapsules
obtained by spray-drying.

A second modification of this process (Figure 4) produces microcapsules by spraying an emulsion with a hot melt composition as the continuous phase into a cooling chamber.  Film-formers useful in this process include natural and synthetic waxes such as mineral waxes, vegetable, animal and Fischer-Tropsch waxes, sometimes modified with synthetic resin materials.

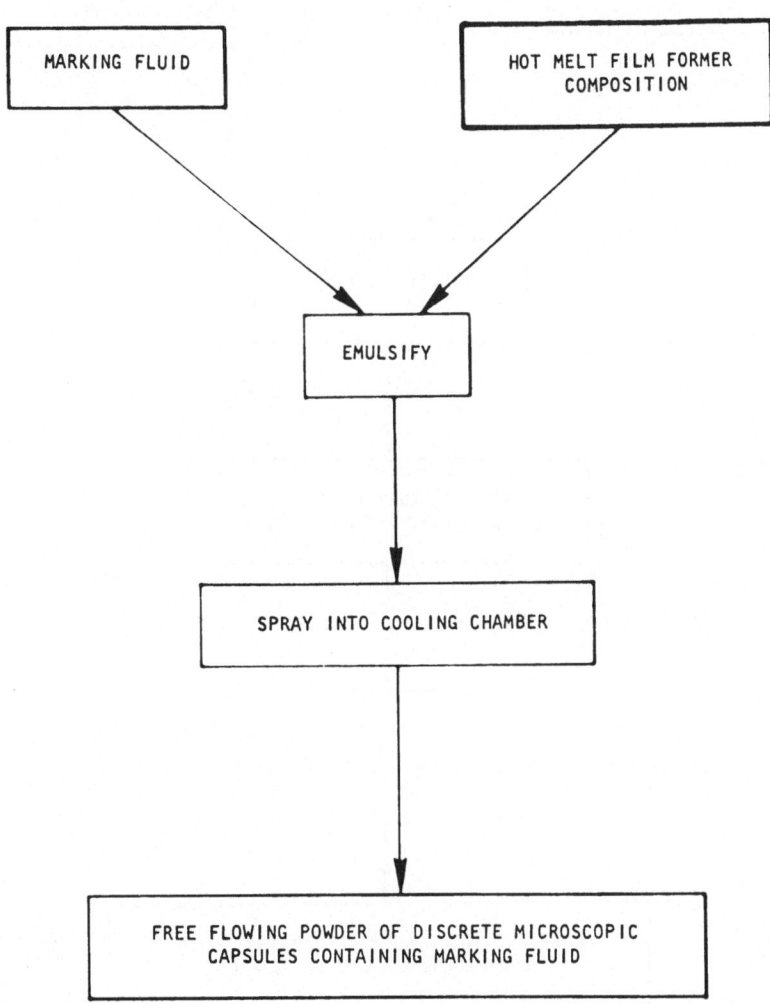

Figure 4.  Microcapsule formation by spray-cooling a hot melt emulsion of marking fluid.

Figure 5 outlines a process for microcapsule formation by condensing a water-soluble resin in the emulsion continuous phase around droplets of marking fluid as the dispersed phase and spray-drying the resultant microcapsule suspension.

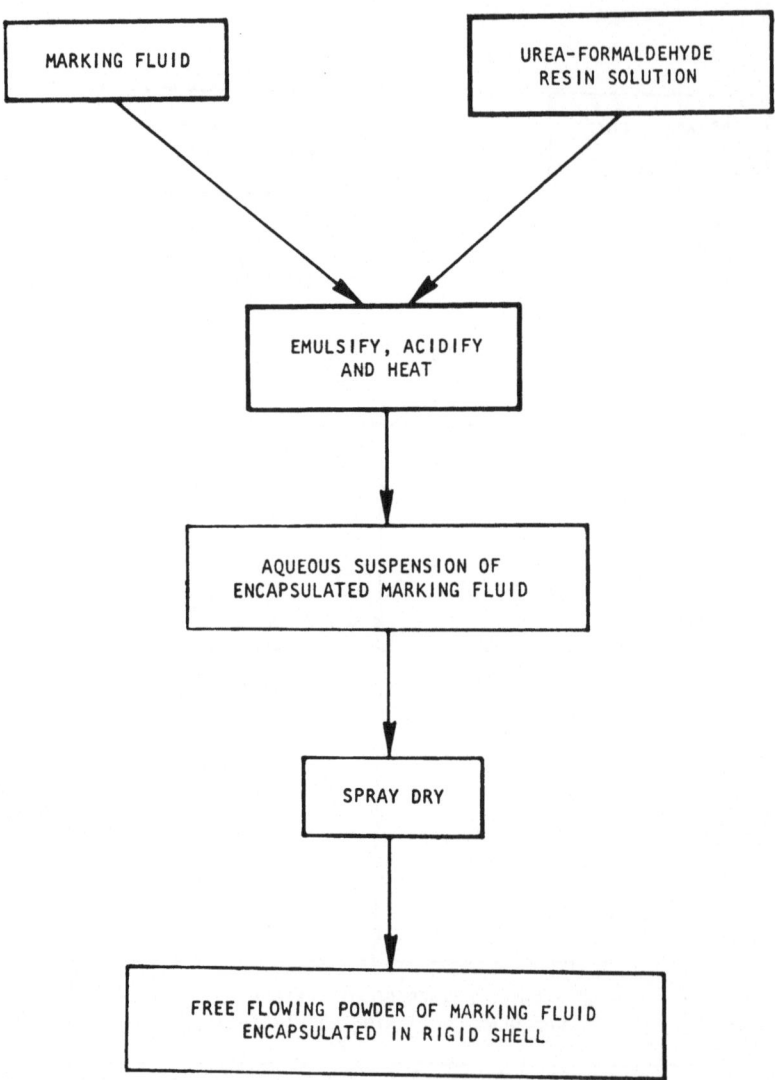

Figure 5. Microcapsule formation by condensation of a water-soluble resin as emulsion continuous phase around liquid core droplets, followed by spray-drying.

Urea-formaldehyde resin is most useful in this process and microcapsules prepared by this means are shown in Figure 6.

It will be apparent that microcapsules prepared according to these examples permit considerable flexibility in the choice of film-formers and marking fluids.

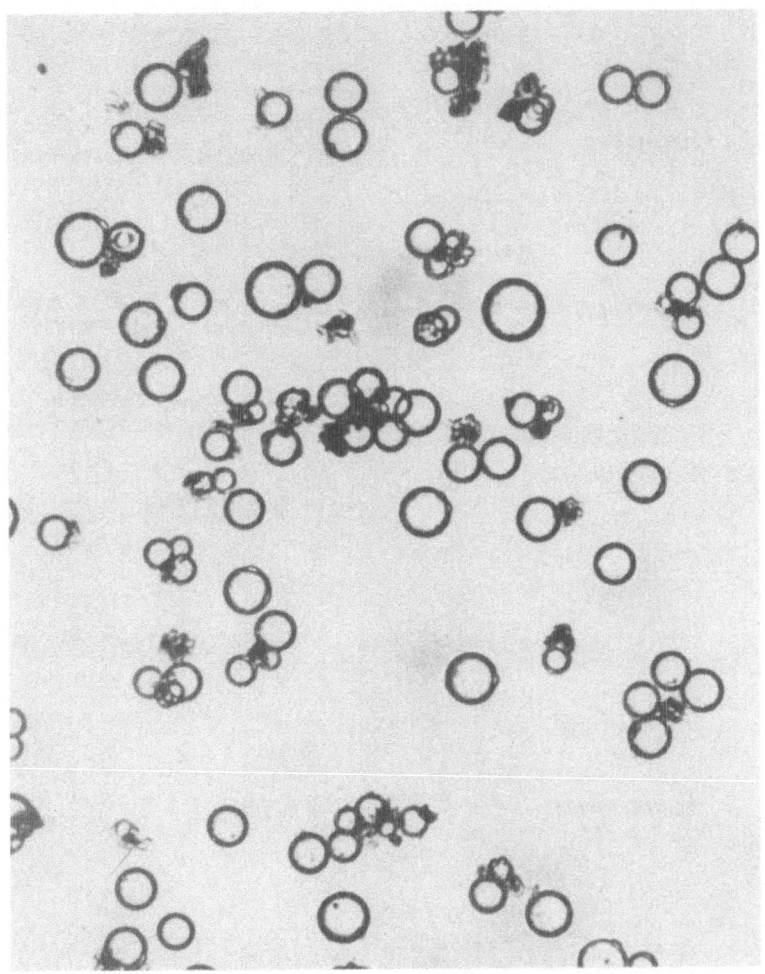

Figure 6. Photomicrograph of urea-formaldehyde microcapsules prepared by condensation and spray-drying.

## Microencapsulation by Interfacial Polycondensation

This process makes use of a modification of known interfacial polycondensation techniques to produce a thin, high molecular weight polymer film as the capsule shell. These techniques are well described in the literature references appended to this paper. Essentially, the process comprises bringing two reactants together at the reaction interface between the emulsion phases where poly-condensation occurs virtually instantaneously to form a thin film

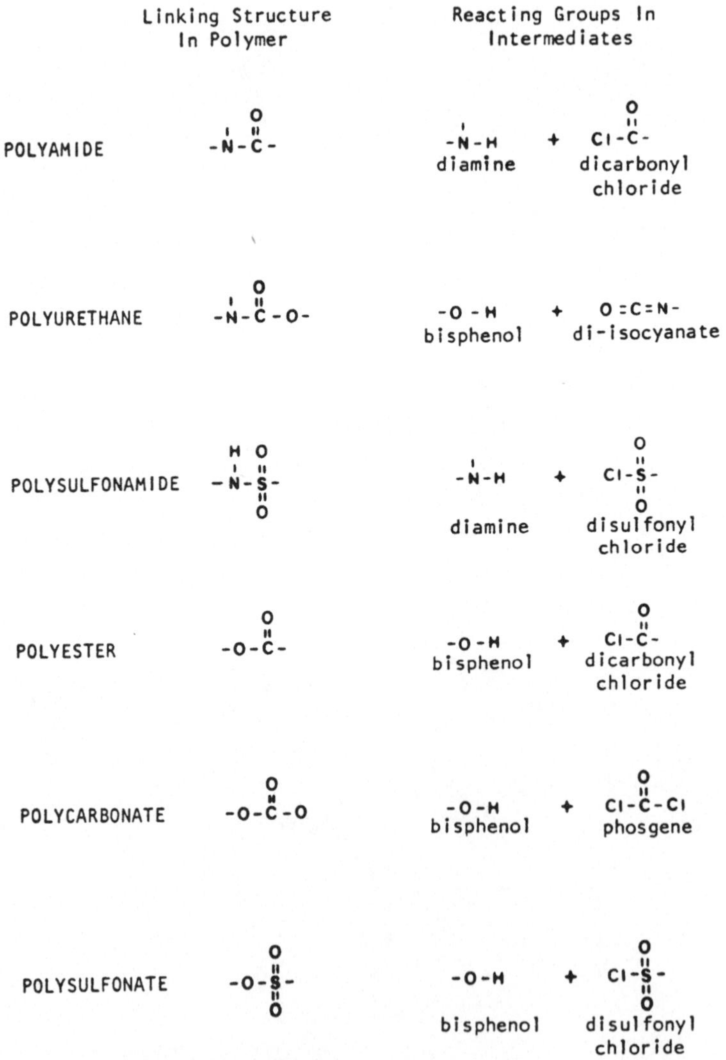

Figure 7. Chemical classes of polymers useful in micro-encapsulation by interfacial polycondensation.

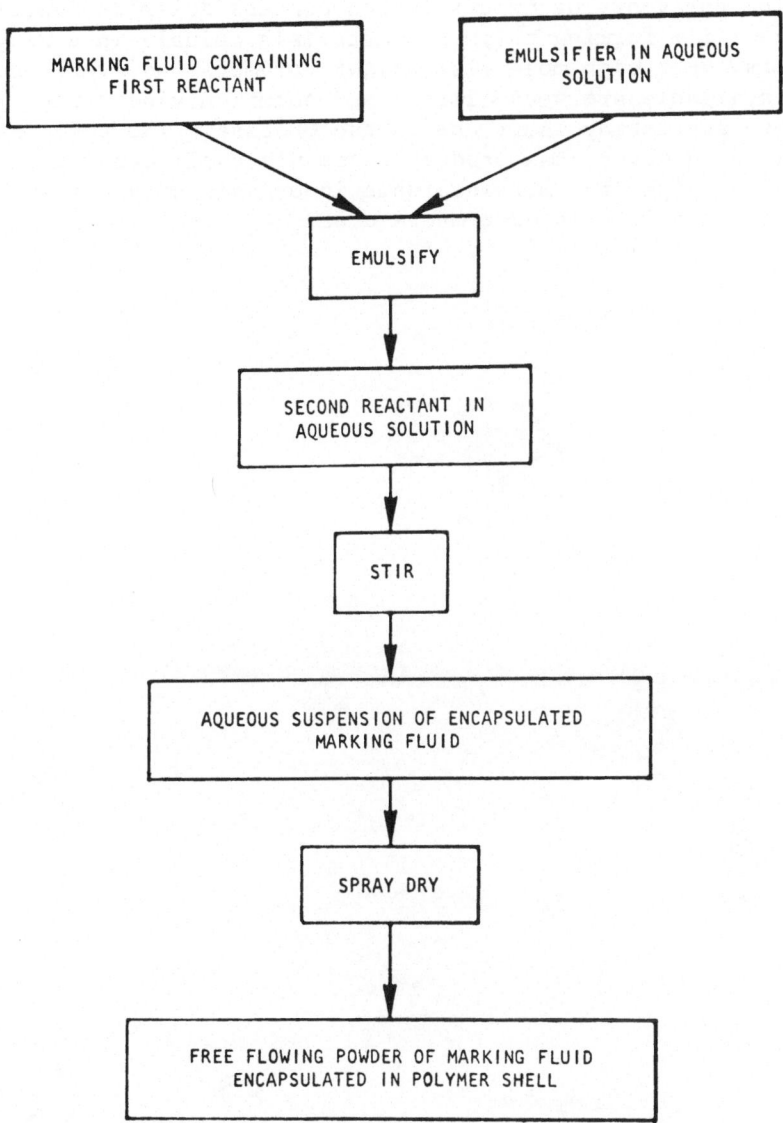

Figure 8. Microcapsule formation by interfacial polycondensation.

insoluble in the parent media of the reactants.  Some classes of
polymer which can be prepared by this technique and which have been
used in encapsulating a variety of materials are shown in Figure 7.

The spray-drying encapsulation process described earlier
utilized film-forming polymeric materials soluble in a range of
solvents.  For high molecular weight polymers, however, the solvents available are very limited and solution viscosities are high,
thereby restricting their use in the process.  The polycondensation
technique, however, can produce a capsule shell consisting of high
molecular weight polymer insoluble in organic solvents and infus-
ible at hot melt coating temperatures.  A particular advantage of

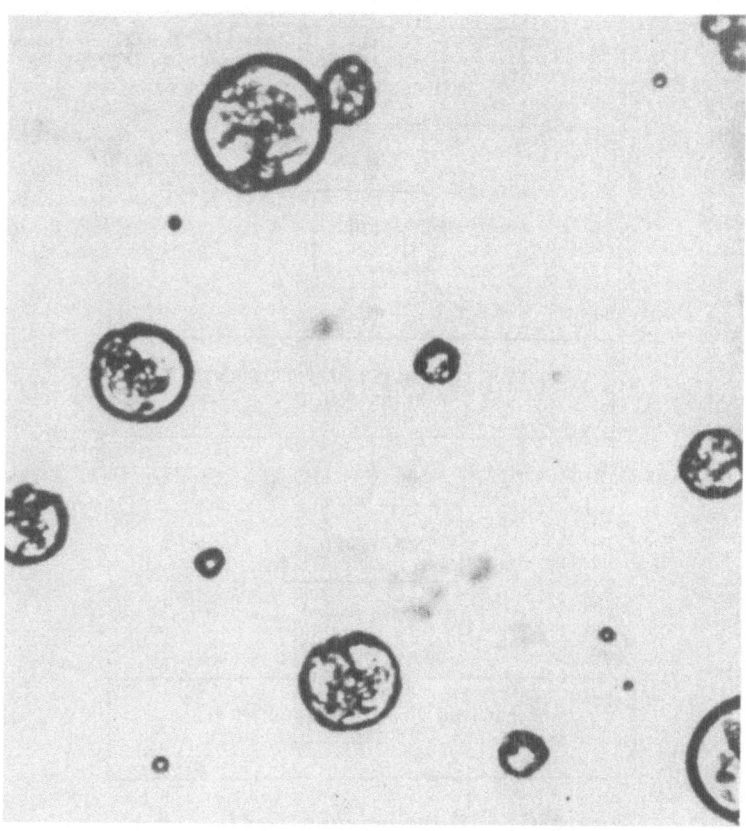

Figure 9.  Photomicrograph of interfacial
polycondensation microcapsules.

the process also is that it provides a method of encapsulating water or water-soluble substances. To control the formation of the capsules, one reactant for the condensation polymer, together with the substance to be encapsulated, is first emulsified in a continuous phase and thereafter additional continuous phase containing the second reactant is added to the emulsion. The polymer shell will then form at the interface of the dispersed substance and encapsulate the material. The sequence of steps in this process is shown in Figure 8.

Figure 9 is a photomicrograph of interfacial polycondensation microcapsules dispersed in water and Figure 10 is an electron photomicrograph of such microcapsules coated on a paper substrate.

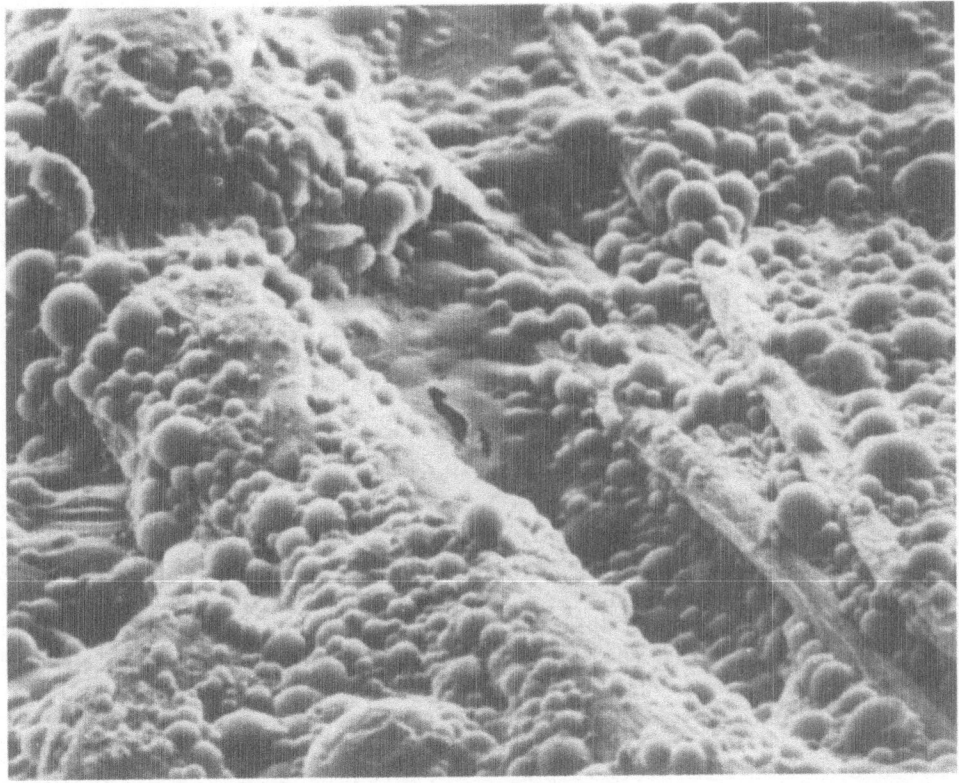

Figure 10. Electron photomicrograph of interfacial polycondensation microcapsules coated on paper.

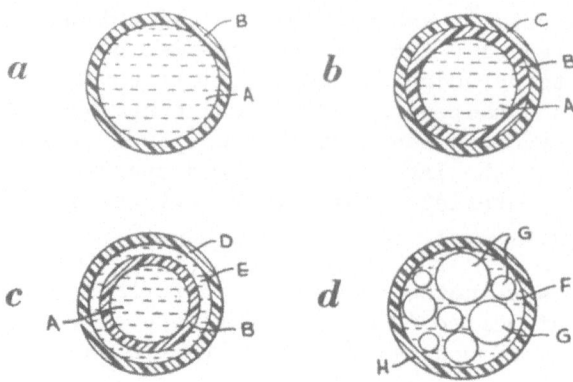

Figure 11.   Interfacial polycondensation microcapsule structures.

Microcapsules having a wide variety of structures can be prepared by this process and some of these are shown in Figure 11.
Figure 11a illustrates a capsule where $\underline{A}$ is the encapsulated material and $\underline{B}$ is a shell of high molecular weight polymer produced by
interfacial polycondensation.  Figure 11b depicts a capsule where
$\underline{A}$ is the encapsulated material and $\underline{B}$ is the shell composed of a
high molecular weight polymer produced by interfacial polyconden-
sation and $\underline{C}$ is a second shell applied by a spray-drying process
or similar technique, or by coating the dry particulate material.
In Figure 11c, $\underline{A}$ is the encapsulated material, $\underline{B}$ is the interfacial
polycondensation shell and $\underline{E}$ represents a second phase which may be
similar to or different from $\underline{A}$.  $\underline{D}$ represents a second condensation
polymer shell which may be the same as or different from $\underline{B}$.  In
Figure 11d, $\underline{G}$ represents the capsules of Figures a, b or c, $\underline{F}$ is a
dispersion medium for capsules $\underline{G}$, and $\underline{H}$ represents an interfacial
polymer shell.

Virtually any material can be microencapsulated by the process
provided reasonable precautions are exercised to avoid selecting
materials which tend to inferfere with the interfacial polycondensation reaction.  Thus, the substances to be microencapsulated can
be gases, liquids or solids which are water-insoluble or water-sol-

uble.  For pressure-sensitive copying systems, it is desirable to
have microcapsule walls which are impermeable to the encapsulated
solvent.  Where pesticides, fertilizers, perfumes or other functional ingredients have been encapsulated, it may be desirable to have
a controlled degree of porosity or permeability in the capsule walls
to allow the slow release of the encapsulated materials.  The versatility of this process allows such control over the final product.
For example, experiments in our laboratories have shown that encapsulated volatile solvents such as toluene and xylene can be contained without measurable loss at temperatures close to their boiling
points for periods in excess of 24 hours.  Alternatively, the capsules can be designed to lose 10%, 20%, 30% or more of encapsulated
ingredient under the same conditions and over the same time period.
Figure 12 shows some data derived for loss of xylene from a range
of microcapsule formulations when held at 110°C over a period of
more than 20 hours.

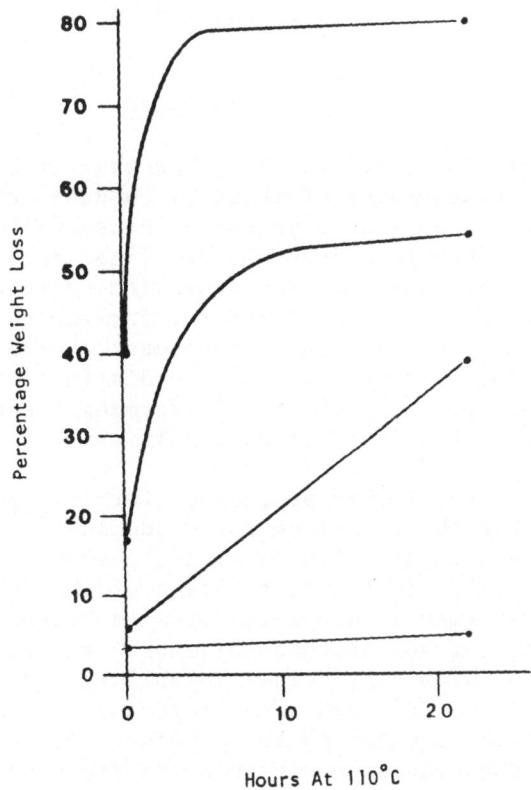

Figure 12.  Loss of xylene from interfacial microcapsules at 110°C.

The efficiency of encapsulation is measured by determining the amount of encapsulated or "free" solvent. The "free" solvent is extracted from the capsule slurry by mixing with an inert extracting solvent. The quantity of "free" solvent in the extracting medium is then measured by either gas or liquid chromatographic techniques. The total solvent in the system is determined by extracting the capsule slurry with a reactive agent which will extract the solvent through the capsule walls, again followed by chromatographic analysis. The ratio of total minus "free" solvent over total solvent is a measure of the encapsulation efficiency. The polycondensation process can be controlled quite readily at an encapsulation efficiency of at least 98%.

Water can also be encapsulated by this process. In one technique, a solution of one reactant in water can be extruded into a solution of the second reactant in a water-immiscible solvent, forming small droplets of water within the solution and instantaneously encasing them in a polymer skin which forms at the interface. A second technique consists of forming a water-in-oil emulsion or dispersion and thereafter adding a solution of the second reactant in oil. The reaction at the interface will encase the water within a polymer shell.

## Dual-Walled Microcapsules

Dual-walled microcapsules in which the wall or shell is constructed of two thicknesses of material, usually of different chemical constitution, have been prepared in several different ways. In fact, one such technique was mentioned earlier in the discussion of the interfacial polycondensation process. In all of these methods, however, the techniques for forming the individual walls are essentially separate and independent from one another. The processes consist of superimposing one distinct wall-forming process upon the product of another wall-forming process, each process requiring control of reaction conditions.

The unique feature of this process of forming dual-walled microcapsules is that the technique for producing the inner wall of the microcapsule automatically initiates the process for forming the outer wall. In the first stage of the process, a proteinaceous film-former is deposited from an aqueous solution around core droplets of non-aqueous solvent in an emulsion as the result of a reaction with a protein-insolubilizing reactant in the core droplets. Acid is released as a by-product of this reaction, lowering the pH of the aqueous emulsion phase. A second hydrophilic colloid in the aqueous phase then undergoes coacervation with the remaining proteinaceous colloid upon reduction in pH to within a predetermined range, and thus an outer skin is formed on top of the first. Such coacervation mechanisms are well documented in the patent literature and elsewhere.

The procedural steps for making dual-walled microcapsules by this method are shown in Figure 13. Following the emulsification step, a thin film or skin can be observed around each droplet on microscopic examination. When a sample of these droplets containing mineral oil, for example, is air-dried on a microscope slide and immersed in toluene, little or no oil is extracted. This con-

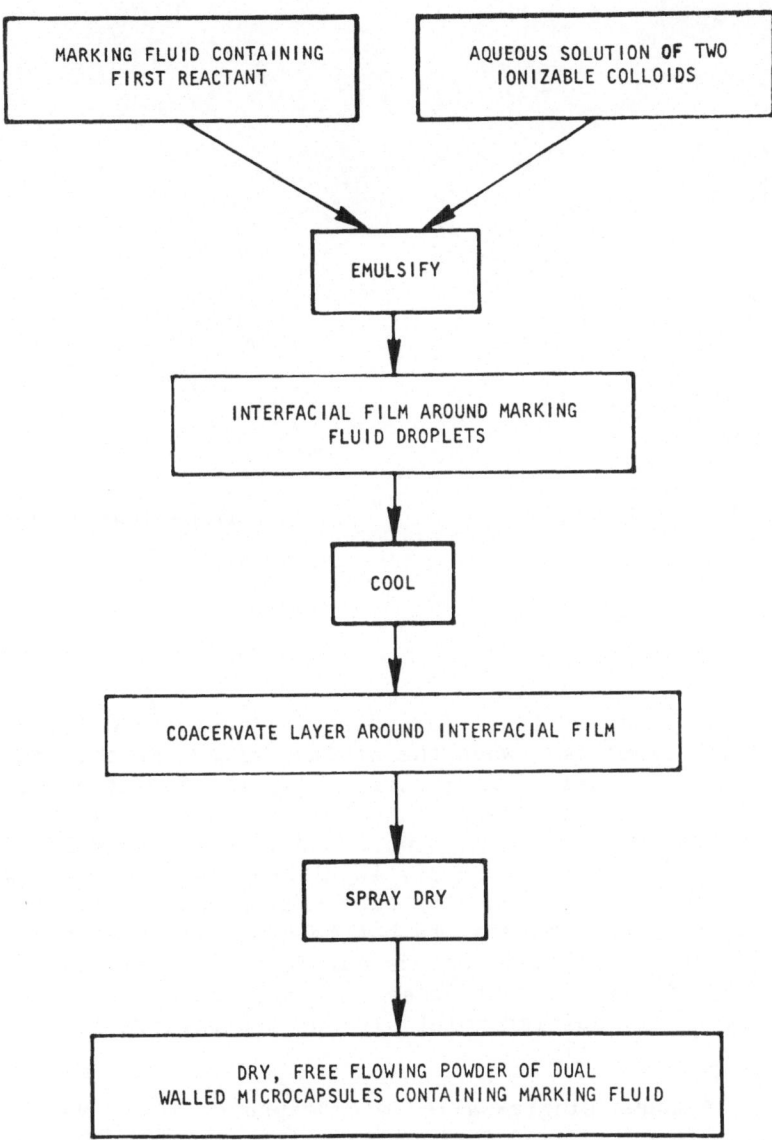

Figure 13. Dual-wall microcapsule formation.

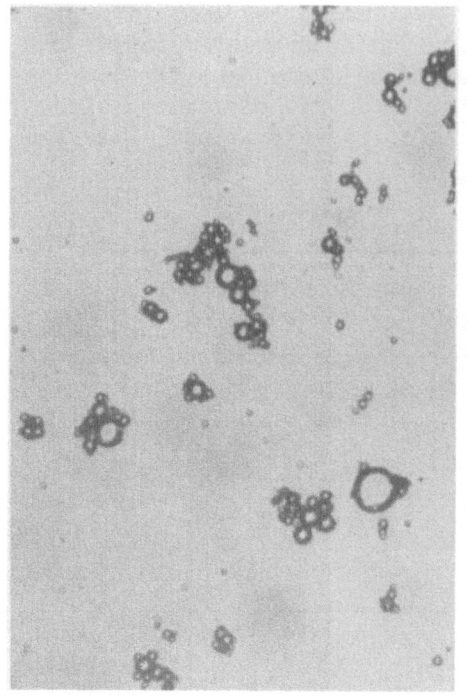 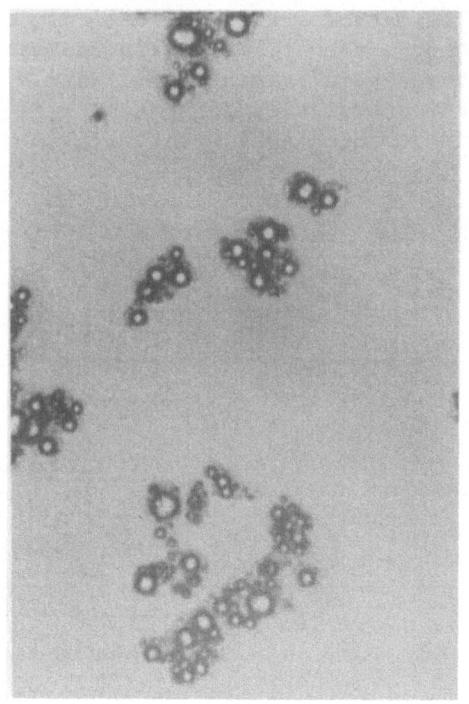

Figure 14.   (a) Single-wall                    (b) Dual-wall

firms that the inner wall has formed as an impermeable layer
around the oil droplets.  When the product after the cooling steps
of the process is examined microscopically, the formation of the
second wall layer can be seen.  This wall has a considerably
greater thickness than the inner wall and is gelatinous in
appearance:  it can readily be distinguished from the inner wall
under the microscope.  Samples of such microcapsules containing
mineral oil have been immersed in hot toluene for up to two hours:
the washed samples released copious quantities of oil under pressure.  Also, similar microcapsules can contain xylene at temperatures close to its boiling point without appreciable loss.

Figure 14 shows single-walled microcapsules after the first
shell-forming reaction, and dual-walled microcapsules after the
coacervation step.

## References

1.  U.S. Patent 3,016,308
2.  U.S. Patent 3,429,827
3.  P.W. Morgan, Soc. of Plastics Engineers J., 15, 485 (1959)
4.  E.L. Wittbecker and P.W. Morgan, J. Polymer Sci., 40, 289 (1959)
5.  P.W. Morgan and S.L. Kwolek, J. Polymer Sci., 40, 289 (1959)
6.  R.G. Beaman, P.W. Morgan, C.R. Koller, E.L.Wittbecker, and
    E.E. Magat, J. Polymer Sci., 40, 329 (1959)
7.  M. Katz, J. Polymer Sci., 40, 337 (1959)
8.  V.E. Shashoua and W.E. Eareckson, J. Polymer Sci., 40, 343 (1959)
9.  C.W. Stephens, J. Polymer Sci., 40, 359 (1959)
10. E.L. Wittbecker and M. Katz, J. Polymer Sci., 40, 367 (1959)
11. J.R. Schaefgen, F.M. Koontz, and R.F. Tietz.  J. Polymer Sci.,
    40, 377 (1959)
12. S.A. Sundet, W.A. Murphey, and S.B. Speck, J. Polymer Sci.,
    40, 389 (1959)
13. W.E. Eareckson, J. Polymer Sci., 40, 399 (1959)
14. D.J. Lyman and S. Lup Jung, J. Polymer Sci., 40, 407 (1959)
15. P.W. Morgan and S.L. Kwolek, J. Polymer Sci., 62, 33 (1962)
16. U.S. Patent 3,578,605

# AIR SUSPENSION ENCAPSULATION OF MOISTURE-SENSITIVE PARTICLES USING AQUEOUS SYSTEMS

Harlan S. Hall, Thomas M. Hinkes

Wisconsin Alumni Research Foundation

7617 Donna Drive, Middleton, Wisconsin  53562

This study was initiated to investigate the feasibility of eliminating the organic solvents in the application of coatings onto solid particles.  While it was anticipated that moisture-sensitive substrates might interact with aqueous coating systems used for encapsulation, it was also realized that the successful utilization of aqueous systems offered economic advantages compared to the use of organic solvents.

For example, if one applies a coating material costing $2.50 per pound from 5% solution in a solvent costing $0.13 per pound, the cost of the solvent can equal the cost of the coating material. If the cost of the coating material is less than $2.50 per pound, the solvent is frequently the largest single cost.

There is also growing concern over solvent emissions and permissible solvents.  While solvent recovery can drastically reduce emissions and frequently reduce solvent costs, such recovery requires capital investment.  If it were possible to avoid the use of solvents, substantial savings would be possible.  Others[1] have described selective coating systems using various ratios of alcohol and water;  however, this study utilized completely aqueous coating systems.

The use of water as the sole solvent has been limited by the fact that many of the materials to be encapsulated are sensitive to water.

The product to be encapsulated can be affected in several ways by an aqueous encapsulation system.  A material may:

dissolve                       e.g. sugar, salt

change states of hydration     e.g. $FeSO_4 \cdot 4H_2O \rightarrow FeSO_4 \cdot 5H_2O$

exhibit instability            e.g. $NaHCO_3 + RCOOH \longrightarrow$
                                    $RCOO^- Na^+ + CO_2 + H_2O$

The pharmaceutical industry has been sugar-coating tablets from aqueous systems for many years; in that process, however, encapsulation of water-sensitive tablets is preceded by the application of a moisture-resistant seal coat such as shellac or cellulose acetate phthalate (CAP) to protect the core. A study of various films used for seal coating has recently been released by Shin-Etsu Chemical Company.[2]

We have used the Wurster Air Suspension Coating Process in our studies because it utilizes very rapid drying kinetics. The process simultaneously applies and dries encapsulating materials onto particles supported by an upward moving airstream (see Fig. 1) resulting in intimate contact between the particles being coated

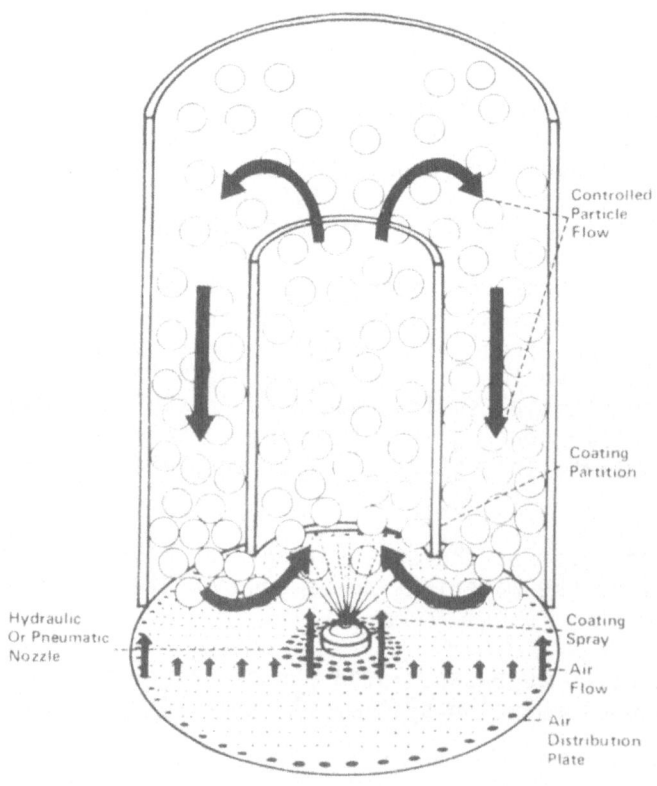

Figure 1

and the drying air.  The movement of particles within the coating
chamber is controlled by the size and distribution of perforations
in the plate, producing a cyclic flow pattern into which the coating material is atomized.  The moving particles cycle past the
nozzle every four to six seconds, receiving an increment of coating
on each pass.  The particles exhibit uniform build-up of coating as
the run progresses.

In the Wurster Process, drying conditions are a function of
the humidity, temperature, and flow volume of the processing air
stream; a significant and unique aspect of this process that
differentiates it from other encapsulating techniques.  The volume
of processing air is determined by the size, shape, and density of
the material being encapsulated; small, low-density particles
require less air flow than large dense particles.

The temperature of the processing air is limited by the sensitivity of either the material being encapsulated or the coating
itself.  A psychrometric chart (see Figure 2) can be used to
determine the drying capacity of the process for aqueous systems.

For example, point 1 on Figure 2 shows the temperature of the

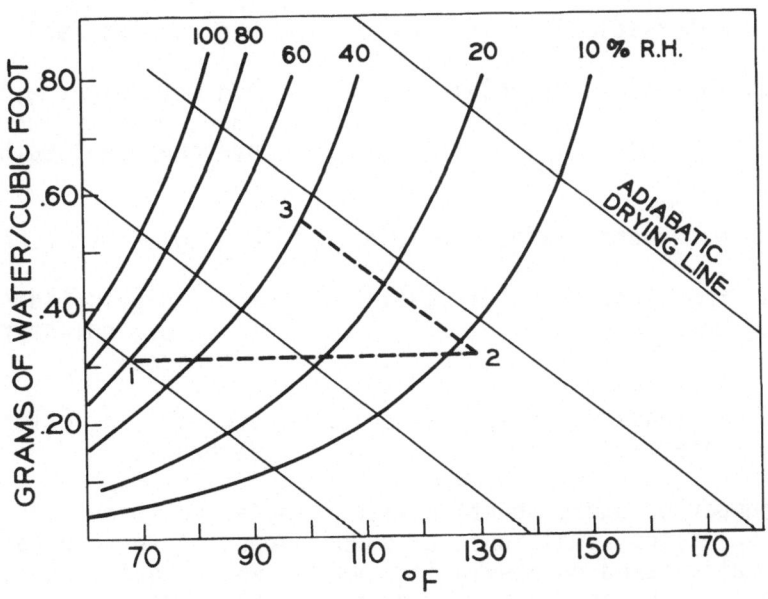

Figure 2

available air at 70°F and 60% relative humidity. When this air is heated to 130°F, its relative humidity is decreased to less than 10%, as shown at point 2. When the aqueous coating solution is applied through the atomizing nozzle, the temperature of the processing air is reduced by evaporative cooling, which takes place along the adiabatic drying line to point 3, 100°F and 40% relative humidity.

The drying capacity of the air is represented in Figure 2 as the vertical difference between points 1 and 3, 0.55 - 0.30, or 0.25 grams of water per cubic foot of air. This weight of water per cubic foot of air multiplied by the number of cubic feet of processing air represents the total drying capacity of the system for these conditions.

The Wurster Process is commonly used for encapsulating and film-coating particles from organic solvents. Pharmaceutical particles and tablets are often encapsulated with cellulose-derived films using solvents such as alcohols, chlorinated hydrocarbons, and ketones. Shellac, waxes, and glycerides have similarly been applied to foodstuffs. More recently the encapsulation of materials soluble in, or sensitive to, the solvent system has been accomplished using the Wurster Process; e.g. warfarin, an anticoagulant rodenticide soluble in many organic solvents, has been encapsulated using an alcohol/chlorinated solvent-based system.

Aqueous coating systems can be grouped into the following categories:

| | |
|---|---|
| 1. Water-soluble compounds | e.g. sugars, salts |
| 2. Water-soluble polymers | e.g. hydroxypropyl cellulose, polyethylene oxide, hydroxypropyl methyl cellulose |
| 3. Water-dispersible colloids | e.g. gums, starches |
| 4. Emulsions of water-insoluble materials | e.g. polyvinylidene chloride, polystyrene butadiene |
| 5. Suspensions of water-insoluble materials | e.g. silica, calcium carbonate |

A number of useful coating materials can be formulated as aqueous solutions, emulsions, or suspensions. A representative list of water-based encapsulating systems which have been successfully applied by the Wurster Process is as follows:

## Cellulose Derivatives

ethyl cellulose  (EC)
methyl cellulose (MC)
hydroxypropyl cellulose (HPC)
cellulose acetate phthalate (CAP)

hydroxypropyl methyl cellulose
(HPMC)
hydroxypropyl methyl cellulose
phthalate (HPMCP)

## Other Materials

| | |
|---|---|
| AEA  Sankyo | hydrolyzed cereal solids |
| Eudragit E | polyvinylidene chloride |
| Carbowax | polystyrene butadiene |
| chitosan | acetylated glycerides |
| acrylics | polyvinyl acetate |
| shellac | carrageenan |
| | |
| clays | whey |
| dextrins | casein |
| gelatins | milk solids |
| starches | soy protein |

Studies with each of these systems have demonstrated that the solvent release characteristics, concentrations, and molecular weights of the polymers, as well as processing conditions and equilibrium moisture content of the films, are all factors which can affect the quality of the encapsulated product.

For this study we selected an aqueous solution and an emulsion system. The water-soluble polymer hydroxypropyl cellulose (HPC) was selected because of its established position in the pharmaceutical industry, and a polyvinylidene chloride (PVDC) emulsion was selected for comparison of aqueous solution and emulsion types of encapsulating systems.

Initial tests were made on placebo tablets at several moisture levels to determine the feasibility of encapsulating from aqueous systems without increasing the moisture content of the final product. Analytical data were obtained for tablets at three moisture levels to determine whether moisture was added during encapsulation with the selected polymer system. In the first column under percent moisture, the control, or uncoated, lactose tablets were encapsulated as received at 3.2 moisture. In the second and third columns the tablets were dried to reduce their moisture content before encapsulating.

| Tablets | Percent Moisture | | |
|---------|------|------|------|
| Uncoated | 3.2 | 2.5 | 1.0 |
| Coated, HPC | 3.1 | 1.4 | 1.0 |
| Coated, PVDC | 2.9 | 1.6 | 1.1 |

The moisture content of the coated tablet is a function of the operating conditions used while encapsulating. The chart shown contains data obtained under normal drying conditions, and indicates that under those conditions little or no moisture was added to the product. When drying conditions are inadequate, the moisture content of the product does increase.

The above data demonstrate that water applied as part of the coating system could be removed by the Wurster Process, but left undetermined whether damage to the core materials occurred. Another series of experiments was conducted to determine the effect of aqueous coating systems on materials known to be sensitive to water. Ascorbic acid and acetylsalicylic acid tablets[3] were selected because both are water-sensitive and both have degradation products readily determined by standard analytical methods.[4]

Decomposition products were determined within ten to fourteen days after encapsulation and again after an accelerated storage cycle of 30 days at room temperature, followed by 30 days at 37°C, followed by 60 days at room temperature. All samples were stored in sealed glass containers.

The Vitamin C tablets used in this study contained 50 mgs ascorbic acid each. They were coated with HPC and analyzed for dehydroascorbic acid, the decomposition product of ascorbic acid. The data show no significant increase in the amount of dehydroascorbic acid as a result of encapsulation with an aqueous system. The analysis is accurate to ± 0.05 mg.

### Decomposition of Vitamin C

(mg. dehydroascorbic acid/50 mg Vitamin C)

| Tablets | 10-14 days | Accel. Storage |
|---------|-----------|----------------|
| Uncoated | 0.19 mg. | 0.12 mg. |
| Coated | 0.15 mg. | 0.17 mg. |

The same coating experiment was conducted using aspirin tablets containing 325 mg. (5 grains) of unstabilized acetylsalicylic acid and analyzed for the decomposition product, salicylic acid. In this test a more distinct pattern is observed which reflects the effect of varying the coating conditions.

### Decomposition of Aspirin

#### (% salicylic acid)

| Tablets | Process air temperature | 10-14 days | Accelerated storage |
|---------|-------------------------|------------|---------------------|
| Uncoated |          | 0.09% | 0.23% |
| Coated, A | 130°F | 0.14% | 0.48% |
| Coated, B | 115°F | 0.12% | 0.18% |
| Coated, C | 110°F | 0.12% | 0.84% |

While all of the above samples surpass the U.S.P. standards for salicylic acid content in aspirin tablets[5], the differences between samples A, B, and C correlate with process temperatures used during encapsulation. These tests indicate that either excessive heat as demonstrated in sample A, or inadequate drying as demonstrated in sample C, are undesirable and contribute to instability.

It is observed in sample B that under properly controlled conditions it is possible to apply aqueous coating systems with a minimum of hydrolysis to the product.

Although this study of aqueous systems has centered on pharmaceutical products, it is apparent that potential areas of application would include:

Encapsulation of seeds

Encapsulation of metals

Encapsulation of food ingredients

Encapsulation of dehydrated products

Encapsulation of flavors and essential oils

Encapsulation of water - reactive ingredients

Uniform application of colorants or wetting agents

The Wurster Process is licensed on a non-exclusive basis by the Wisconsin Alumni Research Foundation (WARF), Madison, Wisconsin, an organization which is authorized to administer and license inventions assigned to it by the University of Wisconsin faculty and staff.

The authors wish to express their appreciation to the WARF management, Dean Dale E. Wurster and Mr. Steve Seely for contributing to the success of this program.

[1]Film-Coating Technology: Dr. C.A. Signorino, Colorcon, Inc., Moyer Boulevard, West Point, Pennsylvania  19486; 1973

[2]Water Sealing of Sugar-Coated Tablets with Pharmacoat 606: Shin-Etsu Chemical Co. (Biddle-Sawyer Corporation, 2 Penn Plaza, New York, New York  10001)

[3]Tablets were supplied by courtesy of Eli Lilly and Company, Indianapolis, Indiana  46206

[4]Analyses were performed by WARF Institute, Madison, Wisconsin. Dehydroascorbic acid: J. Biol. Chem., 147, 399 Salicylic acid: J. Pharm. Sci., 60, 114

[5]U.S.P. - 18, pg. 54, 1970


## DISCUSSION AFTER THE PAPER

Q.    How long does it take to encapsulate particles using the Wurster Process?

A.    The coating of tablets with aqueous systems as part of this study required about 40 minutes.  However, the time varies as a function of the coating level desired and the rate of application.

Q.    How large is a batch?

A.    Most of the development work is done in a 6-inch diameter coating chamber which can be adapted to handle 0.5 to 2 kg of material, depending on bulk density.  Larger units are available which are capable of handling up to 400 kg loads.

Q.    Were the tablets shown in your slides also polished during processing to give the glossy appearance?

A.    No, the tablets were glossy as they came from the processing equipment.  In this case the film material that gave us the gloss was hydroxypropyl methyl cellulose.

Q.    What are the size and shape limitations of the material being encapsulated?

A.    Most commonly, particles in the size range of 150 microns up to about 3/4" are encapsulated, although particles down to 74 microns (200 mesh) can be encapsulated. While it is easiest to process spherical particles, irregular, rough or elongated particles have been successfully encapsulated.

Q.    What limitations are there with regard to the type of materials which can be used as coatings?

A.    The main requirements are that a material be dissolved, emulsified, suspended, or melted so the liquid form can be atomized using hydraulic or pneumatic spray nozzles. This liquid must be dried or cooled on the core material during processing to give a dry film or layer. While this includes a tremendous range of materials, it is necessary to remember that some coatings will be easier to apply than others, and the specific application will narrow the choice of materials.

Q.    How is the Wurster Process distinguished from other encapsulation techniques?

A.    This is a mechanical process as opposed to the chemical and physical methods of other technology. This process is specific for the encapsulation of solid particles and a wide variety of coating materials can be applied.

# PHYSICAL METHODS FOR PREPARING MICROCAPSULES

John T. Goodwin and George R. Somerville

Southwest Research Institute

P.O. Drawer 28510, San Antonio, Texas 78284

## A. INTRODUCTION

Encapsulation is the unique packaging process which is arousing broad interest in many fields. Both liquids and solids may be encapsulated in sizes ranging from a few microns to several thousand microns diameter and in wide variety of shell materials. The capsules may be of use for a number of reasons. These include: (1) protection of reactive materials from their environments prior to use, (2) safe and convenient handling of materials which are otherwise toxic or noxious, (3) means of providing controlled, sustained release of materials following application, and (4) means of handling liquids as solids.

One characteristic which is common to practically all capsules is that the capsule contents are ultimately released. Release mechanisms which may be built into the capsule include thermal release (either by melting the shell or by rupture due to the incorporation of a blowing agent), mechanical rupture, dissolution of the shell, biodegradation of the shell, and controlled permeation or diffusion. Frequently, combinations of these release mechanisms are desirable. Occasionally, there may be a need for capsules which do not lose their contents during their useful life as, for example, where they might be suspended in a fluid stream for metering purposes.

During recent years, encapsulation technology has made great advances with a corresponding increase in interest in capsule utilization. The cost of encapsulation, although not prohibitive in many cases, is a factor in determining feasibility of using this form of packaging. In general, encapsulation is practical in cases where it will do a job which cannot otherwise be done or do the job better, where safety and/or convenience justifies its added cost, where the cost of encapsulation is negligible compared to the value of the encapsulated product, or where encapsulation enhances the value of the product.

## B. APPLICATIONS

Let us look at some of the typical examples of the myriad present and potential uses of capsules. In the propellant field, the encapsulation of highly reactive ingredients might allow their

155

incorporation in propellant formulations as a means of increasing performance. Either liquid or solid ingredients may be incorporated in both liquid and solid propellants. The encapsulation of water for use as a temperature moderator in solid propellants is an attractive application where the use of free water would cause difficulties in the casting of propellant grain or degradation during storage.

Catalysts constitute another class of reactive material for which encapsulation shows advantages. A single package resin system, for example, may be prepared utilizing encapsulated catalysts which may be released under predetermined environmental conditions of temperature, pressure, etc. This technique has been the object of considerable study in space applications for the rigidization of expandable structures and the self sealing of meteoroid punctures. Convenience and extended pot life are other obvious advantages for conventional uses.

Since it is possible to design capsule shells which will release the contained materials either abruptly or slowly under predetermined environmental conditions, wide use may be found in the field of agricultural chemicals. Encapsulated herbicides, for example, may be applied by aerial means without the danger of drift which is carried a considerable distance by air currents as is frequently the case in direct aerial application of the bulk material. The capsules may be designed to remain dormant until conditions promoting plant growth are encountered, i.e., soil moisture and warm atmospheric temperature. Thus, the herbicide would be available on demand.

An agricultural application which has aroused considerable interest involves the encapsulation of amino acids as a ruminant livestock feed additive. In normal feeding of the amino acids, bacteria in the rumen destroy the material before it can be utilized in the intestine. The capsule is designed to effect transruminal passage and provide the desired release in the intestine.

A novel encapsulation development is the preparation of synthetic insect eggs for the rearing of the larvae of beneficial insects for the control of crop predators. Such insects are becoming increasingly important as the predators develop resistance to available insecticides and with the increased hazards of pollution by insecticide residues. Synthetic eggs would have a tremendous cost advantage over natural eggs and would eliminate the necessity for rearing another insect species.

The field of foods and flavors offers another attractive use of capsules. This is particularly true in the case of dehydrated products in which flavors may be released upon hydration.

The pharmaceutical industry, of course, continues to be a major user of capsules, and in recent years, controlled, sustained release medicines have become increasingly important.

In the medical field, the U.S. Public Health Service Hospital at Carville, Louisiana has sponsored the development of pressure sensitive capsules to aid in the rehabilitation of leprosy patients. In advanced stages of the disease, the patients lose the sense of feeling in their extremities and frequently cause tissue damage by applying excessive pressure in manual operations. In many cases, the damage is so severe as to necessitate amputation. The same is true in the fitting of shoes, as deformities often cause severe localized and damaging pressures. Capsules containing dyes or dye precursors, when applied to gloves or socks, provide a visual indication when dangerous pressures are exerted and are a valuable aid in teaching the patient to "feel" again.

This review of typical capsule uses, both current and proposed, represents but a small fraction of possible applications of this unique packaging process.

## C. PROCESSES

For a great many years, most of the interest in this technology was centered in the pharmaceutical area where relatively large gelatin capsules were prepared for oral medication. The familiar two-piece rigid capsule and the so-called sealed or soft gelatin capsule are representative of the pharmaceutical capsules.

The new look, or extension of the old encapsulation technology, has been taking shape during the past several decades with emphasis on the development of capsules much smaller than those which could be made by the older processes and on the use of new shell materials. Two general types of encapsulation processes have evolved—chemical and physical—each having certain advantages over the other. The following comments will be related to the latter type.

Physical encapsulation is perhaps a misnomer, as chemical processes are usually involved. Southwest Research Institute has been quite active in this type of encapsulation work for a number of years, and a brief review of the development work by the Institute will reveal the evolution of various physical processes. In these processes, fluid shell materials are used to form the capsules and are subsequently hardened.

In general, the fluid shell formulation should be essentially immiscible with the material being encapsulated. For example, an aqueous shell formulation would be utilized in the encapsulation of a liquid hydrocarbon. Conversely, a non-aqueous shell material would be used in the encapsulation of water or aqueous solutions. The shell hardening mechanism employed after the capsule has formed is dependent upon the particular shell formulation. The general mechanisms include chemical reaction, cooling, solvent extraction or evaporation, or combinations of these mechanisms. An example of hardening by chemical reaction is the use of aqueous sodium alginate as the shell formulation; the freshly formed capsules may be received in an aqueous calcium chloride bath which rapidly converts the algin to the insoluble calcium salt. The capsules are then rinsed and dried. Molten shell formulations, of course, may be hardened merely by cooling. Latexes are good shell materials when a chemical gelling agent such as sodium alginate is incorporated in the formulation; the alginate provides the initial stability upon being converted to an insoluble salt, after which moisture removal results in a continuous polymeric film. While molten shell systems offer the advantage of simplicity and obviate the need for auxiliary equipment for solvent recovery or drying, higher capsule payloads can be achieved with shell solutions or latexes, as a significant shell shrinkage takes place on drying.

The encapsulation of solid materials is often best accomplished by slurrying finely divided solids in an appropriate liquid vehicle and subsequently encapsulating the slurry as if it were a liquid. Where appropriate, solid materials can be encapsulated in the molten state.

It should be pointed out that proper shell formulation must be achieved to enable encapsulation, to provide capsule stability in the handling and use environment, and to provide the desired release characteristics. The versatility of the physical methods of encapsulation is such that many synthetic polymers, as well as natural gums, waxes and resins, may be used. In most cases, the shell formulation requirements are met by the use of multi-component systems.

The original encapsulation work at the Institute took place about 25 years ago in the development of a method and apparatus for producing relatively large seamless capsules (Figure 1). This figure represents a cross-sectional view of the nozzle apparatus. The fluid shell material enters the device, flows through the annular space, and forms a membrane across a circular orifice located at

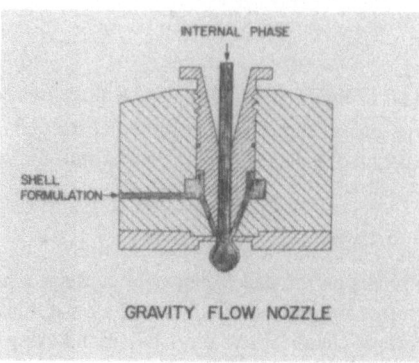

Figure 1

the base of the nozzle. The filler material, immiscible with the fluid shell material, is dropped onto the membrane. As the amount of filler on the membrane builds up, it causes the membrane to distend as shown, and a compound fluid droplet breaks loose from the nozzle. The membrane reforms, and the next capsule begins to take shape. As the fluid capsules fall, surface tension causes them to assume a spherical shape before being caught in an appropriate hardening medium.

Several years after this development, the need arose for seamless capsules having a diameter of about 500 microns. Since the force of gravity is insufficient to form capsules of this size, a device utilizing centrifugal force was designed (Figure 2). The apparatus shown here is representative of several similar centrifugal devices which have been developed. A split flow of fluid shell material is fed into the two grooves of the rotating head where it is held by centrifugal force until overflowing the internal weirs and entering counterbores leading to the individual encapsulating orifices where membranes are formed. The filler material is fed onto a concentrically rotating disc from which droplets of filler material are thrown into the counterbores. When the combined mass of filler and shell materials reaches the point that centrifugal force overcomes the cohesive forces of the shell material, the fluid capsule is released from the orifice and is projected into the hardening medium.

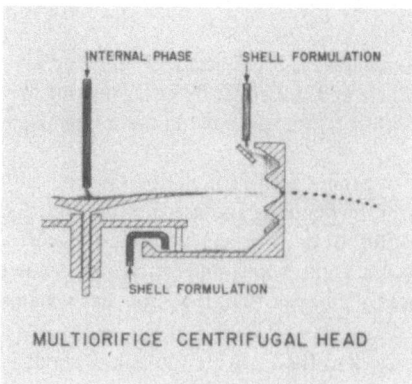

Figure 2

This means, of course, that the rotational speed of the encapsulating head is a determining factor in capsule size.

When producing relatively large capsules, however, the centrifugal force is reduced to the point that the force of gravity becomes significant, and either badly misshapen capsules form or the capsule materials dribble down the outside surface of the head. This problem is overcome by modification of the device (Figure 3) to provide a sloped outer face. Declination of the axis of each orifice is the resultant of the horizontal centrifugal force vector and the vertical gravitational force vector. This configuration permits the production of large, uniform capsules (Figure 4). This is a photograph of the principal element of the device, an 8″ diameter 90-orifice head.

The next figure (Figure 5) represents a simple concentric tube nozzle through which the shell and filler materials are extruded. In effect, such operation forms a fluid rod of the filler encased in a sheath of the fluid shell material, and at a point beyond the nozzle tip, the rod breaks into individual fluid capsules. Although a simple device of this nature enjoys a high throughput rate, capsule uniformity is quite poor. To couple the throughput advantage of the simple extrusion nozzle with the capsule uniformity advantage of the previously described centrifugal devices, the so-called centrifugal extrusion device was developed (Figure 6). As shown in this schematic, the filler is pumped through the inner concentric feed tube, through a seal arrangement, through an inner chamber, and then through radially disposed tubes which penetrate orifices located about the periphery of the rotating head. The fluid shell material is pumped through the annulus of the concentric feed tubes, through a seal arrangement and then through the annuli created by the radial filler tubes in the orifices. As with the simple extrusion nozzle, compound fluid rods of filler and shell are formed and break into individual capsules at some point beyond the periphery of the head. In addition to achieving the objectives of throughput and capsule uniformity, several significant benefits are realized. As a totally enclosed system is involved, temperature control and operation in controlled atmospheres are simplified. Also, volatile fillers may be encapsulated without the losses which are incurred with the previously described open feed disc. In addition to the orifice size, factors influencing capsule size are feed rates and rotational speed of the head. At a given rotational speed, the capsule size increases with feed rate. Increased rotational speed, on the other hand, results in smaller capsules. Thus, it is possible to balance these two factors to achieve the desired size. As a matter of interest, capsules of 350 microns diameter have been produced at a rate of over 300,000 per second per orifice. This compares to about 20 to 30 per second per orifice with the previously described centrifugal device.

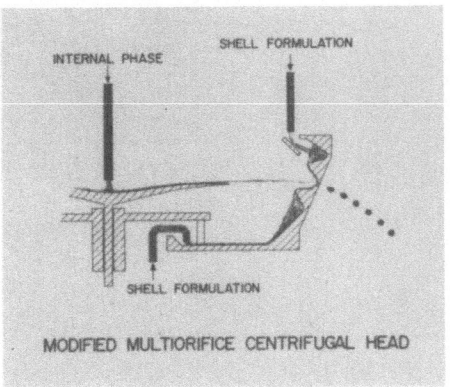

Figure 3

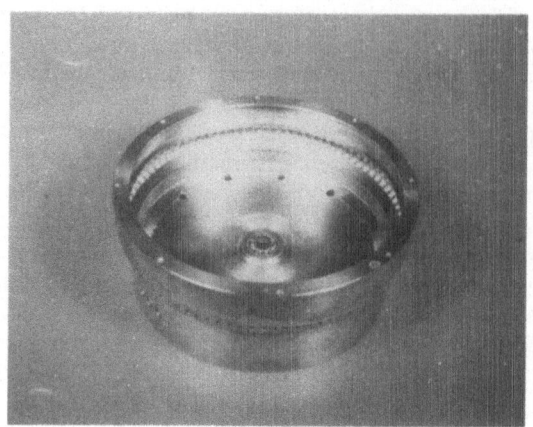

Figure 4

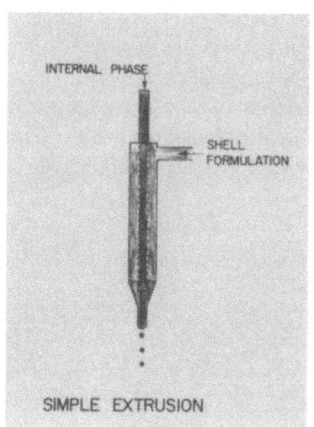

Figure 5

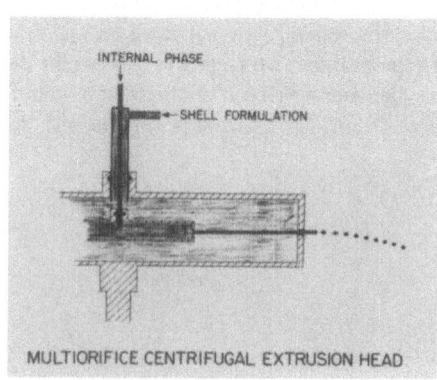

Figure 6

Another device (Figure 7) utilizes a fixed concentric tube extrusion nozzle which is mounted in a duct through which an inert, immiscible carrier fluid flows. The fluid rod of filler and shell materials is attenuated as the carrier fluid velocity increases at the duct convergence, and individual capsules are formed. For any given capsule system, capsule size may be controlled by the nozzle dimensions and by the relative flow rates of the carrier fluid and extruded materials, with the size decreasing with increased carrier fluid flow. This process is particularly attractive in those cases where the fluid shell is quite delicate and breakage may occur on impact with the hardening baths used with the centrifugal devices. As an example of operation of the submerged nozzle device, water or aqueous solutions may be encapsulated using a wax-like hot melt shell formulation. In this case, hot water is the carrier fluid with the temperature in the duct maintained just above the solidification point of the shell. Jacket cooling of the effluent tube is provided to lower the carrier fluid temperature to just below the shell solidification point to effect capsule hardening. The capsules are then removed by screening or other appropriate means, and the carrier fluid is circulated through a heat exchanger to pick up heat removed and is returned to the encapsulation duct.

## D. PILOT PLANT OPERATIONS

Southwest Research Institute is a nonprofit contract research and development organization serving government, industry and individuals in broad fields of science and engineering. Its role in the field of microencapsulation has been oriented primarily toward product development for its sponsors. With regard to capsule manufacturing facilities, until recently the Institute did no manufacturing *per se* other than in support of field tests which were related to sponsored development projects. However, the Institute has now acquired facilities for preparing relatively large quantities of capsules and is able to offer this service to government and industry. This is particularly attractive to organizations which prefer to go through the market development phase without incurring capital equipment or staffing expenditures. The facility also serves to demonstrate the feasibility of scaling up the encapsulation devices which had previously been limited to the laboratory.

This new encapsulation facility utilizes the previously described centrifugal extrusion process. Figure 8 is a view of equipment used to formulate the capsule fill material. In those cases where a slurry is to be encapsulated, sand milling is employed to assure uniformly fine particles and thus

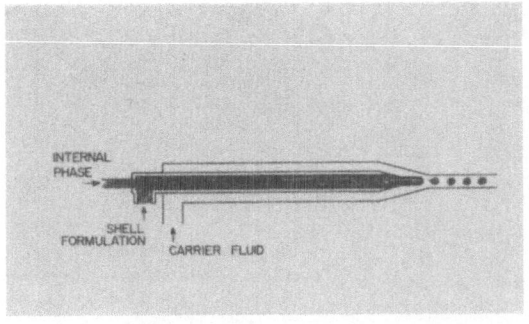

SUBMERGED EXTRUSION NOZZLE

Figure 7

eliminate potential nozzle plugging problems. The fluid shell material is contained in the two kettles shown in Figure 9, one kettle for formulation and one for operation.

The particular encapsulation system depicted in Figure 10 utilizes a molten shell formulation. The encapsulation head, mounted on an elevated platform, projects the capsules to a plastic collecting cone from which they are carried by a vibrating conveyor to a sieve for classification prior to packaging. With a 16-nozzle centrifugal extrusion head, the unit typically operates at a rate of about 500 pounds of capsules per hour.

This encapsulation facility is designed for operation from an isolated control room. Temperatures, pressures, flow rates, etc. are monitored at this point. In addition, a slave stroboscopic light is directed on the rotating encapsulation head, and a closed circuit television system enables constant monitoring of the performance of the individual nozzles of the head.

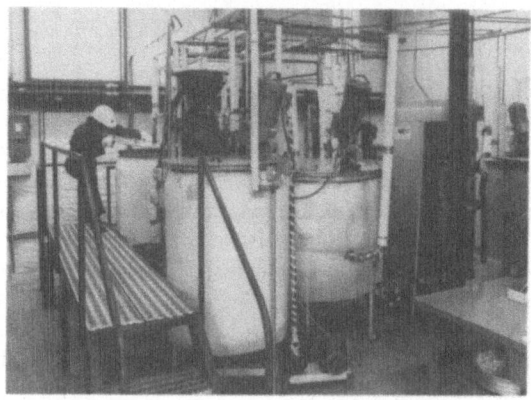

Figure 8

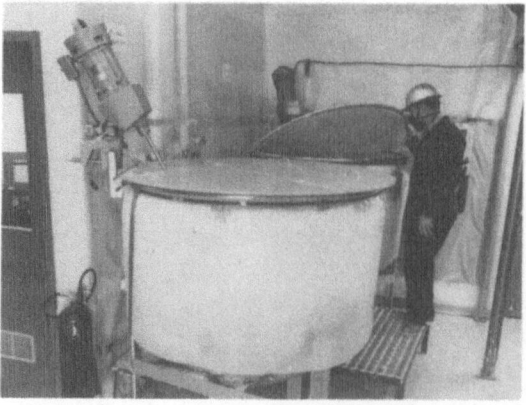

Figure 9

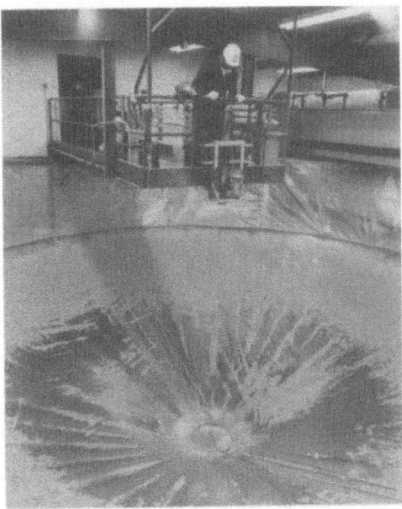

Figure 10

Modification of the general layout of the encapsulation system would be effected for capsules employing shell systems which require liquid hardening baths. In such cases, the encapsulating head would be lowered considerably and the capsule trajectory to the hardening bath reduced to a minimum. Circulation of the bath with capsule removal would be done to provide a continuous process.

Operation of the production facility has effectively demonstrated the reliability of the physical encapsulation method and has confirmed the previous estimates of modest capital equipment expenditures for such a process.

# MICROCAPSULES IN VETERINARY

# MEDICINE: A REGULATORY VIEW

Russell G. Arnold

Bureau of Veterinary Medicine
Food and Drug Administration
Rockville, Maryland    20852

Microencapsulation techniques and processes have been increasingly reported in the literature in a variety of applications.[1-7] Some of these processes have applications in the enhancement of therapeutic medical claims for man and a variety of species of animals. We also see application for use with drugs to promote greater weight gains by the animal consumption of a microencapsulated feed to the economic benefit of the grower.

One of the areas I might mention that has particular interest is the convenience of dosing very large groups of animals once with a drug rather than repeated administration, as this usually involves a greater animal management program. A sustained-release dosage form rather than a conventional dosage form would have a particular use here, and microencapsulation is an approach to sustained-release dosages.

Implants are currently used for sustained-release, and both matrix dissolution and microencapsulation are approaches to this type of drug administration.

In some cases, because the animal systems differ in their activity, selective approaches must be considered for each animal system. In ruminant animals, for example, the digestive system is considerably different from that of other animals in that it is a more complex digestive system. Administration of a drug substance in a formulation may need to be retained in an unaltered form thru the rumen into the abomasum for subsequent dissolution and/or excretion. One way this may be achieved is by a microencapsulation process. Recently, Miller and Gordon[8] of USDA reported

results of a microencapsulated product for the control of fecal
breeding flies by the reduced dissolution of a microencapsulated
pesticide drug with subsequent passage into the manure.  Previous
work with this drug had not achieved favorable results.  The mar-
keted wettable powder form drug was unable to do so because insufficient concentration of drug remained in the feces to kill the
fly larvae.  The microencapsulated drug used in the studies was
able to pass into the feces sufficient active ingredient to obtain
efficacy against two types of fly larvae.

Work reported by Yonchowski of USDA involves the use of
microencapsulation techniques in animal feeds and animal products.
More specifically, the enrichment of unsaturates in the milk fat
content of dairy animals has been reported in Chemical and Engineering News.[9]  The USDA Scientists found that safflower oil prepared
by encapsulation in casein treated with formaldehyde and subsequently placed in the grain ration orally administered to cows, increased
the polyunsaturated linoleic acid content in their milk to an
average 13.6% of total fat as compared with the preexisting 2.7%
unsaturates.  This was achieved by the presence of the casein wall,
which protected the oil from being hydrogenated by micro-organisms
or other processes in the rumen contents of the cattle, thereby
creating the higher unsaturated fat in the milk for human consumption.
Similarly, the USDA Scientists also ran studies where veal calves
were fed milk produced by cows that had been previously fed encapsulated safflower oil.  The milk fat contained 14% linoleic acid.
The calves were not limited in their grain and alfalfa consumption.
Biopsy examination of the calves revealed four times the level of
linoleic acid in their fat compared with the fat of the control
animals.  Microencapsulation thus serves a useful purpose by
delivering a higher quality, more desirable animal product for
human consumption.

Another area of application for microencapsulation would
include stabilization of the active ingredient to achieve a desired
shelf life under expected environmental conditions prior to use.
Approaches to this would be to protect the formulation from heat,
light, oxidation, volatilization, moisture, mechanical stress, or
a combination of these factors.  Medicated Feed Premixes would
particularly benefit from such a technique as they are especially
affected by the above.

Still another area is taste-masking or odor avoidance.  Several
animal species including dogs, cats, and horses can be sensitive
to unpleasant tastes, odors, or aromas associated with the drug
ingredient and/or its related impurities, its degradation products,
the formulation excipients, or combinations of the above.  Additionally, one active ingredient may be protected from the other in
the case of combination drugs.

It is not the scope of this paper to try to elucidate all the currently available techniques that could be used to microencapsulate veterinary drugs. I believe, however, that it would be of interest at this time to direct your attention to the procedure to be used for those of you desiring approval of a new animal drug application for the marketing of microencapsulated product. Here depicted in Table I would be such a sequence. The protocol for studies would be submitted to demonstrate the claim that a microencapsulated product would have a specialized use differing from some other dosage form and that its therapeutic or other medical claims would be delineated. Next, the filing of the investigational new animal drug application would state the types of studies to be conducted and the number of animals to be used. When the exploratory work was conducted and the investigational trials completed, it would be of value to subsequently submit a protocol for a proposed new animal drug application in which proposed studies would be conducted to determine an adequate margin of human and animal safety. The submission should also demonstrate efficacy of the intended microencapsulated drug as administered to the animal. Next, the manufacturing controls would be included in this submission describing the steps and procedures used at each stage for control to the finished dosage form.

When this information is compiled, a new animal drug application would be submitted in triplicate to us for our review. We would review the information in the light of the above-mentioned areas, and a letter concerning our comments would be forthcoming within the statutory limit of 180 days following formal receipt of such application.

When the application has met the requirements of the Food, Drug and Cosmetic Act as implemented by the Regulations, final printed labeling for the product would be requested in writing by the Bureau Director. At that time a Regulation would be circulated within The Administration, and upon receipt of acceptable final printed labeling and promulgation of the regulation, approval of such application would appear in the FEDERAL REGISTER.

Since March 15, 1973 a FEDERAL REGISTER Announcement requires that when a new animal drug application submitted will have a bearing on the environment, an Environmental Analysis Report may be required. This will be a statement delineating the value of the drug, its impact upon the environment, and justification for use in relation to its effect on the environment.

On the next slide, Table II depicts some of our general requirements with regard to a microencapsulation process in the area of manufacturing controls. Here are some of the areas you are going to have to be concerned with when using these processes for a novel dosage form, or dosage form with novel techniques such as you would achieve by a microencapsulation process for a product.

Naturally, in your preparation of this specialized product you will
have your processes controlled, and the limits defined by specifi-
cation.  The particle size range and distribution of the Microcapsules would need to be specified.  In such cases as sustained-
release, taste-masking or other special effects claimed for a
proposed product, sufficient data should be submitted adequately
demonstrating these properties.

Considering some of the general aspects of Good Manufacturing
Practice specified in Section 133 of the Code of Federal Regulations that would have special bearing on these techniques, the
first consideration would be that given to the precautions taken
to prevent electrostatic attraction of dust particulates upon the
microcapsule formulations.  Consideration should be given to
precautions used to prevent cross-contamination of pesticides with
other drugs within the existence of the manufacturing facilities.
With regard to the stability of the product, stability testing to
determine a useful shelf life would be required.  The studies
should include assay for active ingredient integrity, the microcapsule particle size, and disintegration and/or dissolution rate
where applicable.

As discussed earlier, the safety of the wall material as well
as solvents used in the microencapsulation process would have to
be demonstrated by toxicity testing.  Additionally, if the wall
material persists after use, environmental impact considerations
would have to be evaluated to determine whether the product used
could be justified in relation to the subsequent impact on the
environment.  An Environmental Analysis Report will be required
in such instances.

The last statement reiterates point 3 in that specific claims
would have to be substantiated.  The drug content should be expressed as a percentage or other designation and should be indica-
tive of the dosage form; that is, percentages should be expressed
as weight to weight or weight to volume as well as a statement of
the contents of an individual dosage where individual contents are
packaged.  An expiration date will also appear on the label of the
product when data generated by stability indicating assays demonstrate an acceptable shelf life under expected environmental conditions prior to use.  Limits of acceptance of the active drug
content in the formulation should be stipulated as a laboratory
control for the dosage form.  Where sustained-release limits are
proposed for a long-acting or sustained-release product, these
limits and ranges should be stipulated using appropriate statistical
methodology.

For food-producing animals, residue studies are required to
show dissipation of the active ingredient from the carcass to non-
existent or neglible residues as determined by the toxicology of

the drug to assure adequate margin of safety to man and animal.
Adequate residue methodology would be used for detection of drug
residues at the above-determined residue levels.

With regard to submission of this material for a new animal
drug application, there will be cases where the microencapsulation
process will be produced by one company for subsequent formulation
and/or packaging and labeling prior to marketing of the product.
In some cases, a second firm will market the drug and be the
sponsor of a new animal drug application.  The former shall submit
manufacturing data, controls, and other pertinent information in
the form of a master file (MF) to the Food and Drug Administration.
This master file may be referenced by the sponsor of the new animal
drug application by a letter of authorization submitted with the
application.

Overriding all these considerations, of course, is the
economic benefit derived compared with the added cost of product
preparation using a microencapsulation technique.  As the state-
of-the-art increases and technology with these processes expands,
the cost will be reduced.  Additionally, one must keep in mind
that the pharmaceutical elegance of the products should be constant-
ly advancing.  With ecological and environmental considerations
coupled with public interest becoming progressively larger factors
to be considered in the marketing of current products, we would
expect increasing use of microencapsulation techniques for animal
drugs.

Table I.

Sequence for Approval of a
New Animal Drug Application

1.  Protocol for Studies

2.  Filing of INADA
    a.  Safety                     )
    b.  Efficacy                   )  §135 CFR 21
    c.  Manufacturing Controls)

4.  Submission of NADA

5.  Review by the Bureau and by the Administration

6.  Approval of application - FEDERAL REGISTER Announcement-
                              Environmental Analysis Report
                              where applicable.

Table II.

BVM Requirements For New Animal Drug Applications
Using A Microencapsulation Process

1.  Limits of solvents remaining in formulation.

2.  Particle size range and distribution specified.

3.  If sustained-release or taste-masking or other special
    property or effect is claimed, appropriate data adequately
    demonstrating these properties should be submitted.

4.  Good Manufacturing Practice §133 CFR 21.
    a.  What precautions are taken to prevent electrostatic
        attraction of dust to particles after formulation?

    b.  What precautions are used to prevent cross-contamination
        of pesticides or other drugs in the manufacturing facilities?

5.  Stability testing for determination of the shelf life should
    include testing for active ingredient, particle size, etc.

6.  Safety of wall material and solvents used in the microencap-
    sulation process should be demonstrated.  If the wall material
    persists, environmental impact considerations must be evaluated.
    An Environmental Impact Statement may be required in some
    instances.

7.  If specific claims regarding the process to differentiate the
    formulation from competing products such as "sustained-release"
    or "stabilized" or "odor-free" etc. are made, then data must
    be presented to substantiate such claims.

8.  The drug content must be expressed in percent such as w/w or
    w/v.  Limits of acceptance of drug content in the formulation
    should be included as a laboratory control for the finished
    dosage form.  Where sustained-release limits are proposed
    ranges should be defined utilizing appropriate statistical
    methodology.

9.  When microencapsulation processes produced by one company are
    supplied for further formulation, or packaging and labeling,
    or simply marketing by another firm which will be the sponsor
    of a New Animal Drug Application, the microencapsulator shall
    submit manufacturing data, controls, etc. in the form of a
    Master File to FDA.  This Master File may be referenced to
    support a new animal drug application by a letter of
    authorization from the microencapsulator to the sponsor
    and/or FDA.

Question:   Would residue data in food-producing animals need to
            be submitted with a new animal drug application using
            a microencapsulation process?


Answer:     Certainly in the case of a proposed product using a
            new drug substance.  Also, in the case of an existing
            drug, residue data would be needed to show whether
            the metabolism and depletion of drug substance from
            the animal was the same as or different from the
            existing products.  A withdrawal time would be deter-
            mined based on the results of this information.



BIBLIOGRAPHY

1.  Bakan, J.A., and Anderson, J.L., Microencapsulation,
        pp. 384-407, "The Theory and Practice of Industrial
        Pharmacy," Lachman, L., Liberman.

2.  Bell, S.A., Berdick, M., and Holliday, W.M., "Drug
        Blood Levels as Indices in Evaluation of A Sustained-
        Release Aspirin," Journal of New Drugs, Vol. 6, No. 5,
        Sept. - Oct., 1966.

3.  "Semipermeable Aqueous Microcapsules," T.M.S. Chang,
        F.C. Macintosh, and S.G. Mason, Can J. Physiol.
        Pharmacol 44, 115 (1966).

4.  Luzzi, L.A., Zoglio, M.A., and Maulding, H.V. "Preparation
        and Evaluation of the Prolonged Release Properties of
        Nylon Microcapsules," J. Pharm. Sci. Vol. 59, No. 3,
        March, 1970.

5.  Luzzi, L., "Microencapsulation," J. Pharm Sci., Vol. 59,
        No. 10, October, 1970.

6.  Phares, R.E., Sperandio, G.J., "Coating Pharmaceuticals
        by Coacervation," J. Pharm. Sci., Vol. 53, No. 5,
        May, 1964.

7.  Sparks, R.E., "Metabolite Removal in the Artificial Kidney,"
        presented at Microencapsulation Workshop, Hopatcong,
        New Jersey, September, 1968.

8.  R.W. Miller and C.H. Gordon, "Encapsulated Rabon For Larval
    House Fly Control in Cow Manure," Economic Enlomology
    Vol. 65, No. 2, pp. 455-458.

9.  Chemical and Engineering News, July 31, 1972, p. II.

# INDEX